THE FAT GINGER NERD

A WEIGHT LOSS STORY

BRENDAN REID

LONG ECHO
PUBLISHING

CONTENTS

Published by Long Echo Publishing

Contact: https://thefatgingernerd.com

A catalogue record for this book is available from the National Library of New Zealand.

Photo credits: author 2015 portrait by McRobie Studios, author 2021 portrait by Alan Dove Photography.

ISBN 978-0-473-58973-8 (paperback)

ISBN 978-0-473-58974-5 (EPUB)

DISCLAIMER

This book is primarily a memoir. Events of the past, while intended to be portrayed accurately, have been written from the author's perspective; specific details, such as dialogue, may vary from the recollections of others.

The research presented is for informational purposes only, and is not intended as a substitute for personalised medical advice. Please consult with an appropriate health professional before attempting any lifestyle changes such as those discussed in this book, especially if currently taking medication.

To Grandma Reid (1926–2019), who never needed any reason to be proud of me in spite of my issues, beyond simply for being her grandson.

FOREWORD

It's hard, if you haven't been there, to fully grasp what school-yard bullying and society-wide stigma about weight can do to a child. What Brendan does is paint a graphic and sometimes disturbing picture of his childhood world.

This world still exists. Not for him, as an adult who has sent his obesity into long-term remission, but for many, many young people growing up right now.

We haven't solved the problem of being too fat. We've in fact made no progress at all. In fact, it's gotten much, much worse.

So what's the solution?

Should we accept this? That's the fat acceptance movement. And I get that. We should not and cannot continue to persecute people who have problems keeping a healthy weight. It's clearly not an issue of willpower (or lack thereof). It's a problem of a pathological food environment, which disproportionately affects some people.

I get accepting and not blaming. I don't get accepting that we have created a world which will deeply affect not just the physical health, but the mental health and wellbeing of many, many young people.

We do need to figure out some scientific solutions.

What Brendan does in this book is help us understand what it's like to suffer childhood obesity. He opens up that can of worms that reveals how deep being the fat kid runs.

What he also does is take us on his own journey of scientific and practical discovery. It's a journey that he entered with scepticism and a self-experiment just to prove everyone once again wrong. He was fat, and always would be.

Much to his surprise, he has sorted his lifelong weight problem.

This is a journey I have also been on. Not because I was a fat kid, although I did have some issues staying lean, especially in primary school. I think I eventually overcame these more minor body composition issues through nearly obsessive explorations of high-level sport starting with rowing and rugby at high school, leading to running and triathlon into adulthood and culminating with professional triathlon competitions.

I've been more broadly in the field of public health and what keeps people happy and healthy over the course of their life. I spent the first two decades of my academic career focused on the benefits of being physically active.

After all, I had been the poster boy for being physically active for most of my life. I'd sorted out my life by using fitness and exercise. And so could you.

This was also a time when we were finally starting to realise the enormous benefits of being fit and active. A mistake we made in that field, and may still be making, was that being highly active would somehow burn off all that extra fat.

This is an appealing notion, and one which the food industry just loved. There was clear evidence that we were becoming less active, especially our children. And we were getting fatter so we really could solve the obesity problem by prescribing more activity.

While I still study the benefits of being active and how that is important to everyone at every age, what I no longer pronounce is that you can exercise your way into great shape, especially when you have a lifelong problem staying in shape.

What I now know is that the simple calories in and calories out model of obesity was and is wrong. It simplifies a complex biological system into an open loop mechanism. That's not how the human body operates.

A more complex explanation is needed, and the obvious solution follows this explanation.

Brendan introduces you to this science and practice which has turned the world of public health nutrition on its head.

We now understand the control of the sugar in your blood and the hormone insulin that follows, is the important master controller for weight and energy metabolism. We now know that people vary in how their blood sugar and insulin respond to the exact same meal. What one person eats and seemingly has no problem with, can make another fat.

Brendan tells us through his own journey how this all works, and how getting rid of the sugar and ultra-processed food and ultimately adopting a low-carbohydrate eating plan with plenty of healthy fats got him sorted.

I have been privileged to get to know Brendan over the last few years, as his personal journey has turned into a wider journey to help anyone who has had a lifelong battle with their weight and suffered because of it. He is now on a mission to help you and your kids.

If you want to help yourself or others then this is a great read and offers up some of the most important and scientifically accurate information in the field of public health nutrition available.

No, Brendan doesn't have a PhD in public health nutrition. At least not yet; I'm trying to persuade him to enrol. But he does know his stuff. I commend him on what he has achieved here.

I know this started as a cathartic exercise to document his own journey. But it's turned into an important book with the credibility of a boy who defined himself as 'fat', who became a man who eventually found some solutions which you might find useful.

Grant Schofield PhD
Professor of Public Health
Director, Human Potential Centre
Auckland University of Technology

INTRODUCTION

If a man is offered a fact which goes against his instincts, he will scrutinise it closely, and unless the evidence is overwhelming, he will refuse to believe it. If, on the other hand, he is offered something which affords a reason for acting in accordance to his instincts, he will accept it even on the slenderest evidence. The origin of myths is explained in this way.
—Bertrand Russell, Proposed Roads to Freedom, *1918*[1]

1977 was a pretty big year.

Star Wars ruled cinemas everywhere, with honourable mentions to *Smokey and the Bandit*, *Close Encounters of the Third Kind* and *Saturday Night Fever*. In our homes, colour television was still relatively new to many of us, and on those TV screens we were enjoying the likes of *Happy Days*, *M*A*S*H*, *Charlie's Angels* and *The Six Million Dollar Man*.

In music, we were listening to such chart-topping artists as ABBA, AC/DC, the Bee Gees, Debby Boone, David Bowie, the Commodores, the Eagles, ELO, Fleetwood Mac, Foreigner, Billy Joel, Queen, Leo Sayer, Rod Stewart, Donna Summer, Wings and Stevie Wonder. It was also the year in which we lost the King, Elvis Presley.

In technology, the early rise of home computing was under way.

1977 was the year in which Apple Computer was incorporated by the two Steves, Jobs and Wozniak. The Commodore PET computer was first released, as was the Atari 2600 gaming console. On a larger scale, the space probes *Voyager 1* and *Voyager 2* were both launched, and the Space Shuttle *Enterprise*, named after the fictional *USS Enterprise* of *Star Trek* fame, also made its first flight in that year.

And in politics, Gerald Ford was formally succeeded as President of the United States by Jimmy Carter, following the results of the previous year's election. But less well known at the time was another political event that took place that year. An event that would set the tone for the future direction of the eating habits of not just the US, but of much of the Western world, for decades to come.

In February 1977 a US Senate select committee chaired by Senator George McGovern presented a report titled *Dietary Goals for the United States*.[2] Its recommendations included increasing carbohydrate consumption to account for 55% to 60% of energy intake, and reducing overall fat consumption to 30% of energy intake, with saturated fat accounting for 10% only. Dietary cholesterol, sugar and salt were also to be reduced.

These recommendations reflected the emerging wisdom of the time, that fat — particularly saturated fat, through its effects on cholesterol levels — was a primary contributor to heart disease. This viewpoint was not unanimous, with critics such as English physiology professor Dr John Yudkin favouring sugar as the more likely culprit, as per his 1972 book *Pure, White and Deadly*.[3] However, the low-fat movement led by Dr Ancel Keys of the University of Minnesota, on the back of findings from his landmark 1970 Seven Countries study,[4] was gaining the ascendancy.

That observational studies such as Seven Countries — whose power generally extends only to establishing possible correlations, but not actual proof at a causative level — were alone enough for the low-fat idea to gain any traction at all, bears some degree of curiosity on the part of historical observers. As science journalist Gary Taubes described the situation in his 2007 book *Good Calories, Bad Calories*: '*Dietary Goals* took a grab bag of ambiguous studies and speculation

... and then officially bestowed on one interpretation the aura of established fact.'[5]

Recognising the unsettled nature of the wider scientific debate at the time, the National Academy of Sciences (NAS) president Dr Philip Handler challenged the very propriety of the report itself. 'What right,' he asked, 'has the federal government to propose that the American people conduct a vast nutritional experiment, with themselves as subjects, on the strength of so very little evidence that it will do them any good?'[6]

Handler's concerns were echoed by physician and nutritionist Dr Robert Olson of St Louis University, during an exchange with McGovern in July: 'I pleaded in my report and will plead again orally here for more research on the problem before we make announcements to the American public.'[7]

McGovern's mind, however, was already made up. 'Senators don't have the luxury that the research scientist does of waiting until every last shred of evidence is in,' he countered.[8]

The select committee report would go on to form the basis for the United States' official dietary guidelines first released in 1980,[9] which in turn would lead to similar such guidelines being developed in other countries around the world over the course of the 1980s and 1990s, including New Zealand.[10] To this day, the first source of evidence cited for New Zealand's *Eating and Activity Guidelines* (EAGs) is the equivalent dietary guidelines of the United States.[11]

In 1978, the year after that original report was first published, I was born. Thus, my entire life has been lived in the shadow of this prevailing sentiment that, among other things, animal fats are bad for us and that grains are good. And it is at the feet of that very sentiment to which I lay a great deal of the blame for many of the health problems that plagued my life over the years that followed.

I may not be a qualified health expert in the traditional sense. There is no special salutation or title preceding my name, nor do I have any set of fancy letters following it. But here I am all the same, alive and well. That may not sound like much, but once upon a time not so long ago, the chances of that still being the case by now were, shall we say, small.

This would also not be the first field into which I have invested my time without being overly qualified to do so. I have worked in radio, but I never went to broadcasting school. I have taught, but I never went to teacher's college. I have worked in IT, but I don't have a computer science degree.

This book is not about my professional life, however. Perhaps the most remarkable part of that story has just been explained in the previous paragraph. No, this book is about my personal life. A life that, for so long, was a life less than ordinary. A life whose quality and direction was questioned by everyone around me, from family to classmates to teachers to medical professionals to work colleagues. Questions endless, answers few.

This book documents that personal journey of self-discovery. It is a story about how one fat ginger nerd finally fulfilled the simplest of dreams — to just be 'normal' — after half a lifetime of wishing and wondering how to make that possible: by turning his back on the very highest levels of advice that were supposed to have fixed him in the first place, but never did, and as he would later come to learn, never could.

* * *

I used to live next door to a family with an overweight teenage boy, who I would often see shut away in his bedroom as I would walk past on my way home from work. He would spend his afternoons there, playing video games on his big flat-screen TV. I felt terribly sorry for him, knowing exactly what it was like, having once been in the position that he was in now. It was almost like looking at myself from my own earlier years.

He probably believed that his solitary gaming habit was a major contributor to his condition. He possibly believed that he might already have been doing his best to stay healthy, and felt dejected at the prospect that what he was doing was simply not good enough, that he himself was simply not good enough. Maybe you, the reader, possibly feel the same. I know I used to.

This book has been written for those kids of today, who are still like how I used to be. For the families of those kids, whose parents may rightly worry for their future. For the kids of yesteryear whose futures are now on the verge of a most uncomfortable arrival. And for those who despair at the wider situation that our society as a whole now faces: in the timespan of a single generation, the proportion of Kiwi adults with a weight problem has more than doubled, from 28% in 1993[12] to 66.2% in 2020.[13]

The rates of other associated conditions have also skyrocketed during the same period. Estimates of New Zealanders with type 2 diabetes have nearly tripled, from 2% of the population in 1993[14] to 5.9% in 2020.[15] High blood pressure rates have increased from 8% in 1993[16] to 21.4% in 2020.[17] Our nationwide prevalence of chronic metabolic disease has never been greater than it is now.

And in the meantime, many experts continue to claim that the science has long since been settled on these matters; the case closed, the door locked and the key thrown away. Instead, the blame for this collective health crisis lies squarely with the people, for not following their advice sufficiently closely. We all know what we need to be doing. Apparently, we just aren't doing it.

Those, in my opinion, are some pretty broad brush strokes. While it may very well be true for some of us, I certainly don't believe that it applies to us all. At least, not in my own experience. I know I tried my best. I did what I was told, for all the good it did me. Which wasn't much, to say the least.

I was fat long before it was cool, long before it had become normalised to the extent that it has today. The only time in my life that I could ever have been considered a trendsetter, not that I ever wanted to be.

Until, in the space of less than two years, I wasn't fat any more. And what's more, I've never gone back.

That's not something that many people are able to achieve. One study suggests that of those of us who somehow manage to lose as much as 10% of our body weight, the percentage who then go on to maintain that loss for at least a year is around 20%, or one in five.[18]

I wonder how many people there are who have lost more than three times that amount and kept it off for more than five times as long? Probably very few. And yet, for all my lack of professional expertise, I'm somehow one of them.

In no way can I claim to have all of the answers for everyone, of course. I still don't even have all of the answers for myself. But I do seem to have accumulated enough answers for myself to have made a meaningful difference, to have finally been able to alter the course of my life towards something approaching normality for the first time. I can only hope that my own experience provides to others even a fraction of the benefit that it has ultimately provided me.

If I could invent a time machine for the purpose of sending just one thing back to my past, it would be this book. It's like a letter to my younger self, or to that boy who used to live next door. Had I known at that age what I know now, my life could have been so completely different that I cannot even begin to imagine how it might otherwise have turned out.

Time itself, of course, is relentless. It is that inexorable passage of time that gives each new day its own unique value. Every day is precious. Our very mortality gives us every reason to aspire to do what we can to make the best of the time that we each have, to seek to live our lives in as many healthy and meaningful ways as possible.

To work towards improving one's lifestyle patterns takes a very strong commitment to change, stronger than the force of old habits, a radical self-honesty and the ability and willingness to do the research with an open mind that allows one to question previously held beliefs.

May you have the courage to question yours.

1 THE FAT KID

Obese people, particularly those who have made many unsuccessful attempts to lose weight, often have low self-esteem. Obesity or its medical consequences may prevent individuals from doing many activities that they enjoy, resulting in impairment of quality of life. Obese children are often teased at school or feel socially isolated. In some societies, there is a poor perception of obesity by the community at large and obese individuals may experience discrimination in various forms.

—*Stephan Rössner,* Essentials of Human Nutrition, *2017*[1]

FOR THE BENEFIT of readers who haven't been fat before, allow me to give you some idea of what it's like, and why it's possibly one of the most difficult chronic conditions from which a human being can suffer.

Imagine a person with some other issue in their life. Maybe they have relationship problems. Maybe they have financial problems, or mental health problems. Or an addiction of some kind, to gambling or maybe drugs.

Now imagine that they were a stranger to you and you saw them walking down the street in town one day. As a random observer, would you be able to tell that they had this issue? In most cases, probably not. Many people with these sorts of issues become quite adept at hiding them from others. You can escape it, forget about it for a while, at least when you're out in public. No-one needs to know.

But there's no such escape when you're fat. Not ever. When a fat person is seen out and about, everyone notices. Everyone knows that they've got a problem, and in my experience, many people will judge that person for it.

So now imagine seeing that stranger with some other issue in their life, walking down the street with a great big arrow-shaped sign floating above their head, pointing down at them: 'Court case.' 'Behind on payments.' 'Depression.' 'Alcoholic.' Now everybody else knows too, whether that person wants them to know or not.

Finally, imagine being that person, complete with accompanying arrow above your head. For all you know, everyone around you is judging you every time they see you. There's nowhere to run, nowhere to hide, 24 hours a day, 7 days a week, 365 days a year.

That's what it's like to be fat. That's what it was like to be me for more than 30 years.

I've heard it said that the definition of an adult is someone who has stopped growing up and started growing out. I'm not exactly sure how my experience fits into that definition though, because in my case, there were no two separate phases to it at all. For as long as I was growing up, I was also growing out at the same time, right from the beginning.

When I ask my parents what they first noticed about me that suggested I was going to be fat, they tell me it was my appetite. I apparently never objected to a good feed, always eating everything that was put in front of me, and would sometimes borrow from the plates of others as well.

Perhaps it wasn't such a big deal to anyone at first because I was also a keen walker. Some of my pre-school years were spent on a farm; if I found a fence line, I just had to follow it to see where it went. If I found lines on the middle of a road, I just had to follow them too for the same reason. Perhaps if I'd followed those lines for long enough, I never would have grown up ~~to be fat~~ at all.

My father insists that I wasn't always fat, and to be fair, I don't appear to have looked too bad in photos of myself during those early years. But I personally have no memory of ever being told otherwise. My recollection of the first years of primary school is of an experience of two halves. In the classroom, things were generally okay. Outside of the classroom was not such a great time, however, as few of the other kids would have any hesitation in expressing themselves at my expense:

'Fatty Arbuckle.'

'Fats Domino.'

'Fat Albert.'

'Fat Albert and the Cosby kids.'

'Fat Albert *ate* the Cosby kids.'

I didn't even know who some of these characters were, but there was no mistaking the intent behind what was being said.

'Be good,' were the parting words from my parents each and every morning as I headed out the door to primary school. And that was all that I had ever intended to be. So I couldn't help but feel confused at all of the unwanted attention that I was getting. My interpretation of 'being good' meant to be so towards others as well as to myself. But these kids weren't being good at all, at least not to me.

They say sticks and stones may break your bones, but names will never hurt you. But if that were really true, then these names clearly wouldn't have been aimed at me in the first place. And I wouldn't still be able to recall them, all these years later.

So what does a child of that age do when confronted with a problem like this? Why, he tells the teachers about it, of course. And sure, the teachers told off the other kids every now and then. But they soon tired of my constant complaints, and my becoming a nark certainly didn't do my social standing any favours either.

Still, at least I was never beaten up for it. Even then, everyone knew that bruises were something that I could show to someone as proof of what was going on. But words? Words were invisible. They could say whatever they liked whenever the teachers weren't around, and at the end of the day it came down to their word against mine.

The first time it really hit home that I had a problem was when receiving my school report from the end of my second year. One particular line read: 'Needs to do something about his weight problem.'

Ouch. Even the teachers were calling me fat now. They weren't telling off the other kids for being untruthful, they were just telling them off for being mean. So it must be real. I really must be fat.

That only left my parents to turn to for advice, but sadly, like everybody else, even their concerns were exceeded only by their powerlessness. The only suggestion they had for me that I felt sometimes made a difference was to 'suck in your gut', to hold my tummy in whenever I was around other people. I could tell for myself just by looking in the mirror how that could help, but it sure was a lot of work pretending to be something that I wasn't, for so long every day.

The final nail in the coffin for me was a discussion I remember having with another relative of mine. He explained to me the idea of this invisible thing called 'metabolism'. I'd never heard of it before — though to be fair, I was only seven or eight — but basically, some people are just naturally more effective at being skinny than others, he said. You can have a good and fast metabolism, or a slow, bad metabolism; you're either strong with The Force, or you're not. And whatever it is for you, you're stuck with it for life.

So that's settled, then. I'm going to be fat forever, and there's nothing I can do about it.

One has to step back for a moment and understand the world environment that I was growing up in at this time. This was 1980s New Zealand, a time and place where no colour was too much. *Aerobics Oz Style* was all over the television,[2] *Jump Rope for Heart* was the skipping rope exercise campaign in schools,[3] and as far as our diet was concerned, quantity control was all that mattered, particularly when it came to fat.

The established wisdom was that you are what you eat. If you eat fat, you get fat. Fat is full of calories. Weight management is just a matter of energy management: calories in versus calories out. All food contains calories, and all exercise burns calories. Therefore, the solution was to eat less, and move more. Simple. And this all worked for everybody else, so if it doesn't work for me, then there's obviously something wrong with me. If I'm fat, then it has to be my fault.

I used to look down at myself as I walked to and from school — the uniform was Roman sandals in summer, Nomads in winter, shorts all year round — and remember pondering my situation often during that time. Here I am, carrying all this fat. I must be eating too much, because that's what everybody else is saying. So I should be able to just not eat and have my body live off all this fat instead. But why can't I do that? I get hungry, just like everybody else. When I get hungry, I want to eat, just like everybody else. But then, why do I still get hungry when I'm already fat?

It doesn't make sense. It's not fair.

I remember a time when the school organised a fancy dress competition for students. Everyone had to come up with a costume, and there would be a parade through the assembly hall with judges and everything. As an already self-conscious child, this was the last thing I wanted, to be judged for my appearance even more than I already was. Luckily, somebody at the time came up with a manageable idea for me: I could go as a Christmas present. We found a box just big enough for me to climb into, with holes cut out for my arms, legs and neck, then covered the entire outer surface with red and blue wrapping paper. The only thing I won that day was my relief when it was over, but that was enough for me.

One day I was invited by a friend to go fishing and water-skiing with his family at a lake about an hour's drive inland. That sounded interesting to me; I'd never tried anything like that before. But it turned out that I was terrible at both, laughably so in the case of water-skiing. Imagine a fat kid skipping along the water's surface like a stone, legs flailing behind him in unbridled panic. But the worst thing was how hungry I was that day. I must have gone through half of the family's food by myself for morning tea, which they only discovered at lunchtime. It was easily one of the most embarrassing days of my life.

'Dinner dinner dinner dinner, Fat Man.'

I was ashamed of myself. I began to avoid other people so that they wouldn't constantly remind me of my failure. I began to fear and avoid failure itself. I focused more on the things that I was good at — maths, for example — and began trying to get out of things that I wasn't so good at.

But even maths would remind me of myself occasionally. One time in Standard 3 (Year 5) as part of a lesson about statistics, we all got our heights and weights measured and our numbers were put on these two big graphs. My height was somewhere in the middle, no worries. But my weight? Way over there, off to the right. At age nine I was 47kg and easily the heaviest not just in my class, but in my entire year.

'[The fattest girl's name] should be your girlfriend, then the two of you can be fat together.'

As I continued to grow in every direction, my physical capacity began to decline. Where once I wasn't half bad at the high jump and used to finish in the middle of the pack in short sprints, now I was falling further and further behind.

By Standard 4 (Year 6) I had begun to lose touch with most of my original circle of friends as I simply couldn't keep up with them any more. They were a generally active and popular crowd, playing games outside all the time both at school and on weekends. Rugby in winter, cricket in summer. I always loved cricket and still follow it to this day; curiously it's one of the very few activities that I was ever able to enjoy in a social setting ... sometimes.

'Gimme the ball, you geek.'

There was a week-long school camp during that last year of primary school, at which everyone got an award for having accomplished a little something of note, as decided by the teachers. When the award came up for 'Biggest eater', everybody immediately turned and stared at me. Well, of course the fat kid was a shoo-in to collect this one. The likely winner here could not have been more obvious.

So it was quite the shock — even to myself — that it actually went to somebody else. No, the one I got instead was 'Bravest tenter'. We'd all had to spend a minimum of one night during that week sleeping in a tent outside, paired up with somebody else. Except that with an odd number of children, someone was always going to have to go it alone and, naturally, that someone would turn out to be me.

There was no courage involved whatsoever here. 'Saddest tenter' would have been more accurate.

As the drift away from my old friends continued, I would eventually come to make a few new ones. These kids were a bit different. They were kids who read books, big ones without pictures in them. Kids with cool toy collections that we could play with inside. Kids with computers and computer games. Kids who could be themselves, by themselves. I could do that. That suited me just fine.

Of course, trying to forget about a problem doesn't just make it go away. And I knew that even then. But if I was destined to be this way forever, then what difference would it make anyway? Why not try to minimise its impact on a daily basis however I could?

And the problem certainly wasn't going away, no matter how much I wished it would. Around the age of 12, I was being taken to the local hospital for regular appointments with the local dietitian. I don't remember whose idea this was, only that it wasn't mine.

The decade may have changed by now, but the advice hadn't. The dietitian's natural focus was on what I was eating. You are what you eat. If you eat fat, you get fat. Fat has the most calories, so that's what you have to stop eating. Calories in, calories out. Calories, calories, calories.

It was here that I was first introduced to what was being made out to be my new best friend: a diagram on a great big poster on the wall called the *Healthy Food Pyramid*.[4] And look up there, see? Fat is right up at the top. I need to be eating less fat, and I need to be eating more fruits, vegetables and grains that take up that whole bottom section.

Alrighty, then. Let's see what I was actually eating in those days up to this point.

Breakfast was usually a bowl of cereal, drowned in low-fat milk, then with a teaspoon of sugar on top to make the whole thing palatable. If I was still hungry after that — which was most mornings — I was allowed up to two pieces of toast with whatever I wanted on them.

I prepared my own lunch every morning before school, and for many years the lunches for my younger siblings as well. Sandwiches for everybody, a couple of pieces of home baking or sometimes a savoury treat like a cold sausage, and a drink bottle full of fruit juice. Orange mango was the only flavour going, as it was the only flavour everybody liked.

Dinner most nights was fairly straightforward. A typical evening meal would feature mashed potatoes, a couple of other veges (beans, carrots, peas and corn were common), and some meat, usually in the form of sausages, saveloys or mince.

It didn't seem to me like there was much fat to remove from what I was eating anyway, but we tried as best I could. No more cheese on my toast or in sandwiches. Meat to a minimum; no more sausages in the lunchbox. I was already drinking low-fat milk so that was fine. I could also eat as much bread as I wanted because the pyramid said so, and for a while there I would learn to eat the slices dry. No butter at all, obviously; that's the worst kind of fat. Maybe just a smidge of margarine here and there if I was lucky.

Vegetables were historically a bit of a challenge at times, but I did manage to score an important — if accidental — victory, the day I discovered how much more appetising vegetables became with the addition of tomato sauce. The sauce itself was okay of course, since it's made from tomatoes, so that was a nice win-win.

There seemed to be just one problem with all of these changes. I never seemed to stay full for very long. It would only be a couple of hours after each meal that I would start to feel hungry again, and not only did the feeling seem to come around sooner than before, but it would also be a stronger feeling than before. And I still seemed to be gaining weight as well.

Okay, so that's two problems.

The dietitian told me that I needed to eat less overall, to get the calorie count down even further, but that was always going to be difficult with hunger already becoming a more regular issue. So she tried putting me onto these special shakes which were supposed to suppress my appetite. They didn't taste very nice, but I was usually able to finish them eventually. Perhaps that was part of how they were supposed to work. Maybe I wouldn't eat quite so much if I didn't like what I was eating quite so much.

And did they work? Well, sort of. I'd have them in the afternoons and then not want any dinner, but dinner was when I had my vegetables, and I needed to have those too because the pyramid said so. And by the next morning, I would still be hungry again anyway, and the scales were still moving in the wrong direction.

Clearly I still hadn't being trying hard enough to lose this weight, so it was time to get super-serious. Now, I was prescribed a diet of nothing but crackers, cottage cheese and water. Surely that would keep the calories under control?

Whether it did or not, it certainly came at the cost of what little appetite control I had left. This diet was agony. For as long as I was on it, I don't think I was ever not hungry. I would get so hungry that it would hurt, sometimes to the point where I could hardly stand up straight, clutching my cramping stomach in tears from the pain. But it had to be for the best if I wanted to lose weight, because the dietitian said so. These were the experts in their field, after all. And so, somehow, I got through an entire month between appointments doing exactly what I was told.

So I was understandably full of expectation when I went for my next weigh-in, but boy, was I to be disappointed. It turned out that I'd put on two more kilograms that month. Not only was I still getting heavier, but I was getting heavier at an even faster rate than I was before.

Nobody else in the room was happy about that, either. This result was utterly confounding for the dietitian; she was convinced that I hadn't been following the diet, but I really truly had been. Mum was conflicted as well; I could tell by the way she and the dietitian were looking at each other that she wanted to believe me, but I was sure she had her doubts too.

I suppose that from their point of view, such suspicion might have been understandable, but I really wished they had put themselves in my shoes in that moment. Anyone who remembers their own adolescent years will recall how important it was at that age to feel normal, to feel like you belong, like you fit in. Now, as someone of that age who most certainly did not appear normal and as a consequence most definitely did not fit in, I had all the incentive in the world to make this diet work. And yet I couldn't.

In any case, as much as we couldn't agree on why it wasn't working, what was clear to all of us was that it simply wasn't working. Beforehand I was fat, and now ... I was fat, hungry, tired and miserable. The very best official advice had come to nothing. I'm still going to be fat forever, and there's still nothing I can do about it. I'm a failure.

And so finally, I was granted the mercy of parting ways with the dietitian. No point in adding further suffering to existing suffering. The first thing I did when I got home that day was make myself my favourite snack: a raspberry jam and cheese sandwich. And man, that tasted good.

That experience would colour my view of dietitians for the rest of my life. From then on as far as food was concerned, I would try to observe the pyramid only as best as I felt capable of doing, focusing on eating plenty of grains, and as little fat as I could. But to consciously go on a diet? Not a chance. Never again.

* * *

As strongly as I had come to feel about dietitians, there were other people in my world that I would come to despise even more. At least I was only seeing dietitians once a month for maybe half of one year. But physical education (PE) teachers? Once a week, minimum, every year.

Just as dietitians would focus on the calories coming in, the PE teachers were all about the calories going out. It was their job to see as many calories burned as possible every time they saw me and, in return, it was typically my wish to see PE teachers burn every time I saw them.

The problem I had with PE teachers was twofold. Not only could they dispense as much pain and suffering as dietitians, and not only were they permitted to do so more frequently (to the point where a friend and I even dubbed one of them 'Deathbringer' behind his back), but they actually seemed to take pleasure in their work. It was as if they enjoyed making my life a misery. They would act as if their enthusiasm was supposed to be contagious, and that I was wrong to feel bad about whatever new torture they had devised for me that day. Because it was 'all for your own good'. They were all so sure.

The annual cross-country run was as much a particular delight for them as it was particularly difficult for me. In my first year at intermediate school, I tried so hard to keep up with the pack that after no more than a couple of hundred metres, I caught the stitch so badly that I couldn't even stand up straight. They thought I was faking it, and only allowed me to retire when they eventually realised that none of their most serious threats — multiple detentions, after-school stay-behinds, letters to my parents, the works — were going to drive me on.

It wasn't even enough that I was a primary target of theirs during regular PE classes and events. During Form 2 (Year 8) they would also take me out of other classes on Wednesday afternoons and make me run around the block some more, with a handful of other fatties. I was the fattest of them all of course, and likely too the most angry, the most bitter, the most depressed, the most sullen. Not the best sort of outlook on life that one could take into their teens, but it was mine.

There were some small moments of rebellion as a consequence. When we had to write and perform speeches for the annual school speech competition, I refused to make one that year. The teachers put me in front of the class anyway as punishment. When I was happy to do so, they tried to raise the stakes by putting me in front of half the school. I was happy to do that too. The joke was on them: I had nothing to lose. What possible harm to my self-esteem could they do, beyond what my size was already doing for me, every single day?

In the lead-up to that year's cross-country run, I was so determined not to take part, with last year's episode in mind, that I deliberately rolled my ankle by walking around on the outsides of my feet until one finally went a little too far. And it would have worked too, if it wasn't for the rain that postponed the event for a few weeks, by which time my ankle had healed again. In the end I just walked the entire course.

Walking was still something that I could manage, at least most of the time, but even my ability to do that would be put to the test as well. During that year's school camp, the class was sent to climb Little Mount Peel in rural Canterbury, a peak of 1300m. It didn't look that 'little' to me on the day. To prevent the group from becoming too strung out on the track, we were arranged roughly in order of physical ability, with the best of us kept to the back of the pack, and the worst of us — guess who — literally setting the pace for everyone else up front. Gee, no pressure.

The climb through the forest was steep, too steep for me at times, but I was constantly being nagged from the people behind me to keep going. The short break just above the tree line was a huge relief, but soon enough we were soldiering along further up the ridge again, now shrouded in thick cloud which would deny us any perspective of accomplishment that a view would have given us at the top.

Still, I did actually manage to make it to the top that afternoon, though I'm not sure I'll ever understand how. We all got to leave messages in a visitor's book in a hut at the summit; mine was something simple along the lines of 'I can't believe I actually made it', but I would also have included a great deal of swearing if I felt that I could have gotten away with it.

Come high school, I had pretty much worked out how the rest of my life would play out. I already knew that I was going to be fat forever, and there was nothing I could ever do about it, so I began to learn to accept the consequences that would come with that life. I would have few — if any — friends. I would die alone and before my time. If that was truly all I could ever hope for, then so be it. At least I would have a few years of freedom to look forward to. But I still had to survive high school first.

In preparation for my arrival, I combed through a copy of the curriculum and the school rules. There were a few reasons for this: I still wanted to 'be good' to the extent that I could, and as such, I still wanted to avoid getting into trouble for anything unforeseen. But I also wanted to be sure of how much more physical activity lay ahead of me, and what I could do to minimise it as much as possible.

PE classes were said to be compulsory for the first two years; beyond that, the subject was optional. I was pleasantly surprised to discover that neither athletics sports days nor swimming sports days nor cross-country running days were compulsory, they were all just 'strongly recommended'. And detentions could only be issued for disrupting the class to the point where other students were being prevented from going about their learning. This was all good to know.

Not that it mattered much in the beginning. The first athletics sports day rolled around and I simply turned up in my regular uniform, having no intention of taking part since I knew that, according to the rules, I didn't have to. But it turned out that the teachers didn't really care about what 'turds' think (this was a common name for 'third formers', a.k.a. Form 3 students, now Year 9). As far as they were concerned, everyone was taking part in some capacity, and it's detentions for everyone who won't. Because I wasn't dressed to compete, I was sent out to be a helper at various events, timing the sprinters, replacing the high jump bar, raking the pit between long jumps and so on.

It's perhaps worth mentioning at this point that in New Zealand, there is very little ozone layer to speak of. And here I was, a fat, freckled, pasty-white ginger, spending an entire late summer's day outside, against my will, with no sunscreen or hat.

By the time I got home, I'd already advanced beyond both pink and red, and was well on my way to a lovely peeling shade of purple. Mum was as horrified as I was already pained, and I had to take a few days off from school to recover. The only good thing to come out of this experience was that I was able to remind everyone who would listen that this was what happened 'last time', and thankfully, I would never be forced to participate in any day-long annual sporting activities again.

There were a number of ups and downs during those earlier high school years. I was surprised to have enjoyed drama classes more than I'd expected beforehand, though on reflection it made sense. In drama, everyone gets to pretend that they're someone else; in drama, it didn't matter to anyone that I was fat, any more than it mattered in good old maths and science.

On the flip side, there was home economics. I remember one time when we were tested for our ability to prepare a simple plate of meat and vegetables. My veges were well judged for having been boiled into oblivion, but I was marked down for frying the sausages in a pan instead of in the oven, where the fat could be drained away. 'You should know better,' I was told, in a tone that made it sound like: 'You — of *all* people — should know better.'

And of course, there were those two years of compulsory PE classes to get through before I would be completely free. It was a thought that I would cling to throughout that period, getting through each class one day at a time. Every time I did anything, whether it was being picked last for a team or coming last in a race, that would be one less class that I'd ever have to suffer through.

One particular memory stands out from my fourth form year (Year 10), where the class was taking turns at landing a basketball through the hoop inside the gym. Once each of us had made a successful shot, we were allowed to sit down and watch those remaining. By the end I was the last one standing, naturally. No matter how hard I tried with my aim, I just couldn't seem to land it. Even the other kids began to feel sorry for me as they watched on.

When I finally got one in after what felt like an eternity of trying, the class applauded out of pity more than anything else. The teacher was as elated as I was furious. How could such a simple game of elimination turn into something so embarrassing? I didn't ask for any of this. I didn't want any of this. When it came to PE, I was so clearly the weakest link, and I couldn't wait to say goodbye to it forever.

Then came the news at the end of that year. For the fifth form (Year 11) the following year, the curriculum was being changed, and PE was to be made compulsory 'on a trial basis'. And the trial was to last the entire year.

You have *got* to be kidding me.

That year I tried to cut a deal with the teacher on the basis that this change was still only supposed to be a trial. I proposed to him that I would do my honest best in things that I felt I was capable of doing, and in return I would be excused from things that I felt would be overly embarrassing (such as swimming) or even dangerous (such as gymnastics) for me to be attempting. To my surprise, he agreed.

I wouldn't go as far as to say that I enjoyed that year overall, but it was perhaps the least terrible. There seemed to be less of a focus on pure exercise and more about just trying to have fun, mostly through various sporting activities. Like cycling, for example: in one afternoon race around the suburb, I finished 10th out of two combined classes totalling around 50 students.

There was a bit of rugby. I anchored the front row in the scrum, fed the lineouts and made a few tackles. In one game I found myself with the ball on the right wing and with open space in front of me as I lumbered towards the try line. Our actual winger came alongside for the pass, but I wanted so badly to score the try for myself that, by the time I realised that I wouldn't make it and finally passed the ball, the winger had overshot me, and the pass was ruled forward.

In badminton I was part of an unlikely but successful pairing; my partner had tennis experience, so he was naturally strong from the back of the court, and I got to make use of my fast reaction time up at the net. That same reaction time — honed through years of video games — would also serve me reasonably well in table tennis, well enough to earn more than a few angry words from some of my classmates. After all, who wants to be beaten at anything by the fat kid in PE?

There was even some of my old favourite, cricket. In one outdoor game, I remember a friend and I being the last pair to bat for my team. All the jocks ahead of us had been dismissed cheaply while trying to show off to the girls, and while my friend and I scored only a couple of runs between us, we at least managed to ensure that the team batted out our overs.

In another indoor game, my team was chasing. I was last in again, facing the last ball of the game needing four runs for the win. I'd been accidentally eye-gouged earlier in the match in a freak fielding collision, and was barely able to see out of my left eye as it wept blood, but I somehow still managed to drive the final delivery back past the bowler to the long-off boundary for victory. My teammates mobbed me in celebration afterwards in what was — for someone like me — a rare and special moment.

And yes, the teacher that year was true to his word. I was allowed to sit out the swimming, the gymnastics, and anything else where I felt that my participation would have just been a waste of everyone's time. There could have been worse ways to get through my final year of PE.

Well, of course there was. At the end of the fifth form with the sixth (Year 12) looming, guess what happened? That's right, another curriculum change. PE was now being made compulsory again, as another 'trial', for a full fourth year of high school.

I was incensed. Not again? Yes again. For three years I'd done my best within the rules both set officially by the school and then unofficially by negotiation. But it still wasn't enough. Parole for the fat guy: denied.

Well, since this was another 'trial' and not to be set in stone for future years, I could at least do what I could for the fatties that would follow me in those future years: to make this trial fail, even if I myself was still stuck with it. So I resolved to turn up to class every single day in my regular uniform, and refused to participate in each and every class, for the entire year.

My protests were more or less both issued and received in silence throughout that year. But things came to a head just after lunch on the last day of my last year of high school. I turned up as normal, wearing normal, and the teacher decided that she'd try to make an example out of me in front of the class. 'Brendan, I'm sick of your attitude, you haven't done a thing all year, go have yourself a detention.'

'You can't do that,' I replied.

She straightened in surprise, turned and faced me. 'Oh really, and what makes you say that?'

'I have read the school rules,' I said. 'I can only be sent to detention if I'm disrupting the rest of the class. My not taking part in anything has not inspired anyone else to do the same, therefore you can't send me to detention.'

This was fast becoming a game of verbal tennis, and the other students were the spectators. 'Perhaps you'd like to go to the principal's office and tell him that?' she offered.

'Really, I'd like to think the principal knows the rules of his own school, or don't you think so?' The crowd liked that one.

She hesitated. 'Well then, you can sit inside and write some lines.'

Fine by me. She led me inside, and wrote something inane on the whiteboard for me to copy about how senior students should set a good example and whatnot, and left the room to take the rest of the class outside.

I paused to decide what to do next, and made up my mind. Whiteboard be damned, this was my Ahab moment. I let it all out, piling upon the paper the sum of all the rage and hate accumulated across an entire adolescence of humiliation and misery. Every vile, obscenity-laden thought that came to mind was written and aimed at every PE teacher in the world. They had extracted all the calories out of me that they could, and despite both their efforts and mine, I was still easily the fattest guy that anyone knew.

The teacher returned at the end of the hour, and at first seemed impressed that I had written so much in that time. Two nearly full sides of an A4 page. Then she began to read it, and her face fell dramatically. Then she broke down completely as she tried to explain that she was just trying to do her job. 'If you don't learn to exercise,' she spluttered, 'you could die!'

'It's my life,' was all I could offer in response. I didn't enjoy that I was making her upset like this, but I didn't enjoy being told over and over to do something that clearly wasn't working for me, either. Regardless of what she was saying, I was well and truly beyond caring at this point. Finally she just tossed the piece of paper back at me in teary-eyed resignation and walked out.

I took the paper with me to my final class of the year, which happened to be physics. I showed it to my friends who wanted to know what had happened. They began passing it around the class, and it eventually caught the attention of the physics teacher, whose eyebrows rose as he assessed its contents for himself. 'This is awfully vitriolic, Brendan,' he remarked simply.

Such was the strength of my conviction by this time. How many fat kids had these PE teachers ever been able to turn around? They thought they knew it all, but none of them had been able to do a damned thing for me, or anyone else like me.

All throughout my schooling years, the attitudes had always been the same. Everyone else is normal because they watch their calories and they exercise, so if you're fat, it's your fault because you're either greedy or lazy, or both. But I didn't feel consciously greedy, I only felt hungry. Was that so unreasonable? I'd always tried to follow the food pyramid to some degree or another, seemingly more closely than most others my age. And I certainly didn't feel lazy; that last year aside, I'd behaved myself the whole time.

And it wasn't like I was completely sedentary out of school, either. I walked or cycled to school and back every day, often into a fierce northwest headwind on the way home. For a couple of summers I cycled across town on the weekends to pick raspberries at a local orchard for a little pocket money. I had a weekly paper round for a few years after school as well.

I also played plenty of backyard cricket with the neighbourhood kids on the tennis court next door to home. The far fence was four runs, six if hit on the full, six and out if the ball was hit over the fence on the full, so as not to waste too much time trying to retrieve the ball

all afternoon. I scored a century there once, but I equally enjoyed firing down my looping leg-spinners.

Yet it seemed all for nothing.

I left high school at the age of 17, weighing a full 120kg. I was still fat, but at least I was finally free. But as for exercise and gyms? Not a chance. Never again.

2 THE ESCAPE

I believe there is something in [fairy tales] that does what singing does to words. They have transformational capabilities, in the way melody can transform mood. They can't transform your actual situation, but they can transform your experience of it. We don't create a fantasy world to escape reality, we create it to be able to stay. I believe we have always done this, used images to stand and understand what otherwise would be intolerable.
—*Lynda Barry,* What It Is, *2008*[1]

LET'S take a moment here for some perspective.

Yes, there's no denying that growing up fat was a far from pleasant experience for me. But my childhood wasn't always that bad all the time. Over the years I realised that things would generally only tend to go wrong either whenever I had to go outside, or whenever I had to talk to people. So naturally, I would adapt by doing less and less of both. After all, they can't hurt you if they can't see you. Inside good, outside bad.

It was while hidden away safely inside that I began to explore some of the available options for things to do with my time, very much a set of circumstances through which I was essentially learning how to live within my physical means. And it didn't take long to figure things out from there. Books don't push you around. The TV doesn't laugh at you. Computers don't call you names.

The last of those three habits would turn out to be the one that I would embrace the most strongly. From behind a myriad of computers and computer desks I can recall many happier times over the years, even if they were mostly by myself or occasionally with the rare contemporary that I might come to call a friend.

Most of those good times, more specifically, came about through video games. When I look back, it's not hard to understand how one could be so easily drawn into such virtual worlds, when one feels so roundly rejected by the real one. In helping me to get through the bad times, games in effect, became my coping mechanism. Games were my escape.

I've been a gamer of sorts for at least as long as I've been fat. I probably haven't played as many different games as a more typical gamer might have, though. I tend to be fairly loyal with the few games that I do play, often sticking with them for years at a time.

In my experience, gamers make excellent problem solvers. After all, what is a video game but a pixelated puzzle, an imaginary construct, with problems to solve within a given set of rules?

First comes learning those rules, simply understanding the aim of the game, and how to play the game, for example reading the manual, learning the controls. Then comes testing your abilities within those rules through practice of the game. And finally, testing the rules themselves; not to the point of outright cheating or hacking, but looking for loopholes, ways to compound the overlapping effects of certain rules, or to reduce your exposure to certain other rules, to really maximise your success through more creative approaches in gameplay.

Learning how to play video games was harder when I was younger and the internet wasn't really yet a thing, as I was limited to just whatever ideas I could figure out for myself, and maybe what I might read about a game in the occasional magazine. But these days just about every game of note — both new and old — has its own online community fanbase, whose members discuss the game amongst themselves on forums, exchanging ideas, the pros and cons of various strategies, ways to get better.

Generally speaking, when someone figures out something in a game that enables them to improve at that game, they will incorporate it into their strategy, whether it's part of the official advice or not. I like that about gamers: most aren't afraid to try something new if they think it could bring them more success. It doesn't matter so much where the idea may come from, they will simply assess the idea on its own merits.

Over the years I picked up on more than a few ideas for various games that I've played, that I was able to incorporate into my own style. Some of these things I would never have figured out for myself, if not for the power of free exchange of information between people with shared motivations and common goals.

This chapter covers my experiences with a selection of games that I enjoyed for extended periods throughout my life, what I learned from each of them, and how they would help shape my brain into something capable of eventually embracing certain other concepts in the real world. The idea here is that if you can understand the lessons of this chapter, you're probably capable of taking on board the later ideas to come.

You don't have to be a gamer to read this chapter, but it possibly helps.

* * *

The first computer that I ever wanted was an Amiga. This would have been around 1986, I suppose, when I first saw the ad on TV. I don't remember much about it, except that there was this great big wall of bright pixelated art that someone was standing and looking at. The wall art included a large eye that blinked, and then the pixels all leapt out at the person standing nearby. For a young, impressionable — and don't forget, fat — kid like me, I just had to have one.

It wasn't going to happen though, not for a while anyway. My parents were pretty straight up about it, to their credit. They simply couldn't afford one. And even if they could, it would be a lot to spend just on me when I was one of three kids with a fourth on the way. How fair would that have been to the others? Even I could understand that.

So it was quite a surprise during the May school holidays of 1987, when one day Dad brought inside from the boot of the car in the garage, a large box-shaped something wrapped in a brown blanket. I flung the blanket open and inside was … a Commodore 64?

He and Mum explained that it was 'the next model down from an Amiga', and that they'd bought it second hand. The keyboard came with a manual, four games each on their own cassette, a cassette deck for loading them, two joysticks for playing them, and about a dozen assorted issues of *Compute!* magazine for further reading. No monitor was included, but we could connect it to Mum and Dad's TV that they usually kept in their bedroom. As long as I behaved myself, of course.

Of those four games, one of them — *Frogger 64* — proved never to work, but the other three — *Congo Bongo*, *Bruce Lee*, and *Ghostbusters* — saw plenty of action over the next few years. Bruce Lee was probably the most fun for the family as it was the only one that allowed for two players simultaneously, and is also the only one of the three that I still enjoy an occasional round of today. But the game with the most strategy of the three was certainly *Ghostbusters*.[2]

The first aim of *Ghostbusters* was actually to turn a profit. You started the game with a loan from the city of $10,000, with which you could buy one from a range of four different vehicles — one of them being the famous hearse from the movie — and purchase various additional items of equipment to further help with catching ghosts as they appeared around the city, each of which earned a few hundred dollars per successful catch.

Once under way, the game itself ran on a timer of sorts, represented as 'PK energy', and you had until the city's PKE levels maxed out to earn more than the $10,000 that you'd started the game with. Every missed ghost would add more to the PKE total, effectively a time penalty, so catching as many ghosts as possible was important to give yourself as much time as possible to make your money back and maybe even a profit.

In the earliest stages, it was important not to waste time wandering the streets aimlessly while waiting for the next alert about a new ghost in need of busting. Better to take a quick trip back to the station headquarters to restock on traps during those quiet moments. There would be fewer of them as the game progressed.

Once PKE had reached a certain level, there was a chance that the Marshmallow Man himself could spontaneously form and stomp his way through an entire city block. The only way to stop him doing damage when he formed was to quickly deploy the 'ghost bait' item. Each successful baiting of the Marshmallow Man earned an instant $2000 reward, while each failure cost you $4000. This very clearly meant that the ghost bait within the list of gear options at the start of the game was an essential purchase. Without it, there would never be any chance of making enough money in time. Lesson learned: in trying to achieve a goal, some tools are objectively more helpful than others.

Upon reaching the PKE limit, the game had three possible endings:

1. If you don't make enough money to pay back the loan, the city is destroyed and your ghostbusting business is foreclosed. Game over.
2. If you do manage to earn a profit, you are granted a shot at sneaking two out of an allowable three men past the Marshmallow Man, seen dancing outside of the entrance to the Temple of Zuul. If you fail to get two men past the Marshmallow Man, the city is destroyed. Game over.
3. If you make a profit and manage to get two men past the Marshmallow Man, they make their way to the top of the Temple of Zuul where they cross their streams aimed at the temple, closing the portal and saving the city. Victory!

Making a profit — regardless of the final outcome — also

presented you at the very end of the game with a specially generated 'account number' that you could enter in the future, to start again with the amount of money earned on this play-through, rather than the default $10,000. This was an ingenious save-game type system that didn't actually require any game data to be saved; just enter your name and the account number provided last time, and start off with more money next time. Now you could purchase a better car and/or more/better gear, but the difficulty was effectively increased as well, since you now had to earn even more in order to profit.

Ghostbusters was probably the first computer game I ever played where I recognised that I actually wasn't half bad at it. I soon learned that the cheapest car — the 'compact' vehicle — was rubbish, as it was slow and couldn't hold all the equipment I wanted, so I usually started with the hearse by default if I didn't have an account number handy. With a bit more starting money I preferred the stationwagon option, as it both was faster and carried more gear than the hearse.

It wasn't always a straight switch-up in the progression, however. The fourth 'high performance' vehicle was super-fast, but almost too fast, as I would find myself sometimes overshooting ghosts while travelling the streets, and it would ironically take more time to try again to catch them. That, plus the fact that this car couldn't hold as much gear as the others, meant constant trips back to headquarters to restock, which took further time away from actually catching ghosts. This provided another important lesson: the most expensive option isn't necessarily always the best.

The highest amount that I remember ever being able to make in the game was about $62,000, which took maybe a couple of years of practice, on and off. To make that amount I needed the wagon with just about everything attached, and was catching pretty much every ghost that came my way, barring no more than one or two mistakes throughout the game. No wasted motion, every second counted.

I remember reading a magazine article about the game at some point, where people had submitted their account numbers to the magazine to prove how much money they were able to make. The highest I'd read was something like $58,000, so I must have been doing all right. If practice doesn't make perfect, it at least takes you pretty close.

* * *

Epithets such as 'nerd' are not typically cast about without some fair degree of justification. In my case, it probably began as a consequence of my relative success inside the classroom, success which I would come to cling to ever more tightly over the years, to compensate for my general troubles outside of it.

And yet, as much as I enjoyed the likes of maths and science in my primary school years, one other boy in my class enjoyed them even more; his scores typically had the edge on mine, more often than not. We became good friends, however, through our common interests like Transformers, for example. And as my family was still a year away from acquiring our Commodore 64, his computer — an Acorn BBC Model B+ — was the very first computer that I ever learned to use, back in 1986.

The two machines would be comparable to each other in terms of their hardware capabilities, but his collection of games was far larger than mine would be for a long time. Many of them were more complex and required more keyboard controls than I was comfortable with at that time as well. So when I played, I tended to stick to games with the fewest controls, like *Vortex*. But I was just as happy to watch him play other more complex games, like *Repton 3*, *Citadel*, and, most of all, *Elite*.[3]

Elite is an absolute landmark in gaming. One of the first truly three-dimensional games ever made, with its wireframe vector graphics, it was first released for the Beeb in 1984 and swiftly became one of the all-time classics of not just that platform, but others in future years as well. Around 1992 or 1993 I would buy a second-hand boxed copy of the game for my C64, for which I had also bought a disk drive by that time. This version was one of two that I spent many, many years playing.

Elite was a space-based trading and combat simulator set across a series of procedurally generated galaxies of 256 planets each. The overall aim was to advance your pilot's combat rating from an initial rank of Harmless, and working your way through the likes of Mostly Harmless, Poor, Average, Above Average, Competent, Dangerous, Deadly, and finally to Elite itself. This was achieved through destroying enough enemy ships, thousands of them over time. To be able to quickly dispatch multiple enemies required a bit of quality gear though, which in turn meant that when starting out, the first order of business was to succeed in business itself, to make enough money to then buy the gear needed to properly compete in combat.

So the initial focus needed to be on trading, and that meant understanding the in-game market, recognising trends in supply versus demand, buying low and selling high, and finding trade routes that would offer maximum profit, not just in terms of the money made from the trading itself, but also minimising the costs of transport. Like fuel, for starters, and maybe some defensive weapons like missiles and energy bombs, for a little protection while travelling.

Since prices were fixed according to each planet's economy type, it didn't take too long to figure out the most efficient ways of making money. Find two planets in close proximity to each other, one a rich industrial planet, the other a poor agricultural one. Buy computers and machinery from the rich industrial planet and sell them at the poor agricultural one, then buy food and liquor from the poor agricultural and sell it back at the rich industrial. The closer together these planets were, the less spent on fuel. The more peaceful the governments on these planets were, the safer the surrounding space was from pirates.

The money made would allow for various gear upgrades to your ship, particularly to your lasers which would make a big difference when switching to combat later. Other useful improvements included a cargo bay expansion to enable your ship to carry more trade commodities, an extra energy unit to improve your ship's passive shield and energy recharge rate, and a docking computer to automate the process of docking at space stations, the art of which required some solid piloting skills without one.

For its day, the game possessed an incredible depth and complexity. By this time I was capable of managing all of the keyboard controls, and gradually worked my way through to purchasing all of the various ship upgrades until I had everything that I would ever need. Then the game really started to take off, with combat becoming the long-term focus.

From here on out, the game became more of an outright grind for combat rating, as money became less of a factor. Instead of looking for two peaceful planets with opposing economies, I was now looking for two warring planets with opposing economies. This would ensure a steady supply of targets that would help advance my kill count, and still provide loot that I could sell at whichever station would offer me the most cash for it. Well, I still needed to restock on fuel and ammunition every now and then, so why not?

It might come as a surprise to learn that my combat rating only ever made it as far as Dangerous, but to be fair, that was only on the C64 version. The other version of the game that I played for at least as long was the Acorn RISC OS version, at high school for the first few years but later at home as well, once I'd inherited one of the school's machines as they were being phased out there. That version of the game had much better graphics, and used a combination of keyboard and mouse controls which felt far more engaging than keyboard alone. On that version I made it as far as Deadly.

So in spite of playing the game pretty solidly for about a decade, I never actually reached that exalted status of Elite, but I like to imagine that I might have made it had I stuck to the same version over the years.

More than anything else, the lesson that *Elite* taught me was the value of patience. Some of the loftiest goals imaginable require no small degree of effort over an extended period of time. There would be good days and bad days over the course of the journey, but along the way, it's worth remembering that every single step counts.

* * *

My first exposure to IBM-compatible PCs wasn't until 1989, when I made a new friend who had just joined the school that year. His PC was an XT machine, running MS-DOS 3.2 on 256 KB of RAM, with a 10 MB hard drive. Its main weakness though was the green screen monitor with no graphics capability whatsoever.

This was clearly a business machine of its day, not meant for gaming at all. But that only made the challenge of finding games capable of running on such a machine that much more interesting. He and I spent many an afternoon enjoying classic text-based games such as *Rogue*, *Kroz* and *Second Conflict*.

It wasn't until 1993, however, that I was able to play PC games on a daily basis. This was accomplished through an emulator — an application for one type of computer that allows it to run software intended for another type — on the Acorn RISC OS machines we had at high school. For the first time we were able to enjoy PC games with CGA graphics like *Dark Designs* or *Pharaoh's Tomb*, but there was still appreciation for the old text-based titles as well.

Begin was another one of those older titles,[4] a turn-based strategy game from the 1980s set in the *Star Trek* universe in the time of the original series, where you could choose to play for any one of four factions: the Federation, the Klingons, the Romulans and the Orion Pirates. You could then choose your opposing faction from the remaining three, and you could also choose the number of ships for both sides (up to eight each), as well as their types, from small birds of prey right up to dreadnoughts.

I always played the Federation. Given the option, I almost always play who I perceive to be the 'good guys' in any game. My opponents were usually either the Klingons or the Romulans; the ships of the Orion Pirates were often too fast to catch once they chose to retreat.

The difficulty was effectively set by the number of ships defined for each side. Of course to begin with, I would start with a full complement of eight Federation ships against a single Klingon or Romulan cruiser. This was so easy I hardly had to do a thing, as the other ships would quickly destroy the lone opponent for me.

However, such lopsided affairs always resulted in my getting a terrible score — less than zero, even — with an assessment such as 'you couldn't command a garbage scow.' What did I need to do to improve my score?

My friend and I soon worked out that the score was derived not just from the success or failure of the encounter, but for the difficulty we would set for ourselves at the start. We began experimenting with fewer ships on our side and more on the other, and while our scores would improve slightly, it was never by much.

So one day we tried the most difficult scenario we could possibly make: a single ship against eight opponents. This might as well have been our very own version of the Kobayashi Maru, *Star Trek*'s famous no-win scenario. I certainly believed it at the time.

My first tactic was just to try to see how long I could last. I would turn my ship around and plot a course in the opposite direction from the enemy fleet. There was no sense in closing into phaser range, as their combined firepower would easily annihilate me, so it had to be a ranged battle with torpedoes.

But even with torpedoes alone it was rough. They would fire theirs almost as a collective volley, and they would always impact my ship at almost exactly the same time, punching a big hole in one of my shield banks. The next volley would typically see major structural damage and crew casualties. If that wasn't quite enough to finish my ship off entirely, the third volley most certainly was.

What frustrated me at this point was the fact that whenever my ship was hit, it was always hit in the same place. I had other shield banks, but somehow the enemies were able to strike the same spot with every volley. How was this happening?

Eventually we worked it all out between the two of us. Imagine a beach ball with six different-coloured vertical stripes. Each stripe corresponds to a different shield bank for your ship, numbered in a clockwise fashion from 1 to 6. When my ship was getting hit, it was always getting hit on either shield bank 3 or 4. This was because I was always facing away from my enemies at the moment of impact.

So the solution here was to instruct the ship to spin on its vertical axis at just the right time by just the right amount, for the next incoming volley to impact on a different shield bank, instead of the same one that had been hit previously. By getting this just right six times in a row, it meant that all six shield banks would each take a separate torpedo volley, and there was usually just enough time between hits for each shield bank to passively recharge.

This gave me the time I needed to pick off the enemy ships one by one with my own torpedoes, stopping only to pivot my ship to properly catch and absorb the next volley. I didn't need to destroy the enemy ships completely at first, but just damage each of them enough to disable their weapon systems to reduce the incoming damage, and thus give me a little tactical margin for error a little more quickly.

Once all of the enemies had been disabled, it was straightforward for me to turn around and close into phaser range for the kill. With their weapon systems down, they still wouldn't be able to respond.

The game would take a very long time to complete, but with this tactic we were successfully able to defeat eight enemy ships with just a single ship of our own, the most difficult scenario possible in the game. Our scores were nice and high after that.

The lesson from *Begin* was simply one in creative thinking: even if you don't have much to work with, making the best possible use of what you have can still make an important difference.

* * *

In 1990 in my first year of intermediate school, I found a new friend who owned one of the very computers that I had originally wanted for myself a few years earlier: an Amiga. And it was everything I had dreamed it would be. The graphics, the sounds ... they were as good as anything found at the video arcade down the road, another place where we would often spend our time (and money) after school as well.

In addition to his enthusiasm for his computer, he was also an avid reader of science fiction and fantasy novels by a variety of authors. Many a time would I find myself listening intently as he would describe some scenario from whatever book or game that he happened to be currently enjoying.

I myself was never into reading much fiction while growing up. To the dismay of all of my English teachers, I preferred non-fiction instead. I used to wander aimlessly through encyclopaedias like people today might browse Wikipedia on the internet. However, when my friend learned of a new Amiga game being released in 1992 based on Frank Herbert's classic novel *Dune*,[5] he was so excited that even I found it hard not to get excited for him.

Like *Elite* years earlier, the game seemed way over my head, so I was quite content to just sit back and watch him play. The visuals — many inspired, if not outright borrowed from the David Lynch movie — were rich and beautiful, and the music so hauntingly evocative of the desert setting that the whole experience sticks in my mind to this day. Rarely had watching someone else playing a video game ever been so enjoyable.

Dune was a point-and-click role-playing strategy and adventure game, and the role played was that of the main character from the novel, the young Paul Atreides. The aim was to explore the planet Arrakis upon which your family had recently arrived, make friends with the various local Fremen tribes, and build your forces in various ways towards an eventual confrontation with the evil Harkonnen family also stationed on the planet.

The game's beginnings were very easy, your dialogue with various supporting characters practically telling you where to go and what to do next. But over time the game's direction becomes less clear, and for a while you're left to do more or less what you like. During that time we'd generally focus on exploration and mining, accumulating stockpiles of spice that the Emperor would regularly request of us throughout the game.

It was really only once the Harkonnens started attacking Atreides territory that things would start to become problematic. Some of the Fremen tribes now needed to be trained in combat, but switching tribes like this meant less spice coming in, and the Emperor's demands were always insatiable, ever increasing. As was often said in the book: the spice must flow.

There were also only a finite number of Fremen tribes to be found in the game, and on top of that, any tribes caught at a sietch — a Fremen settlement — that was captured by the Harkonnens were no longer available to control, effectively becoming Harkonnen prisoners unless more Fremen were sent to take the sietch back and free their brethren.

I remember the struggles we faced in the early attempts at playing through, trying to train individual tribes in combat but then losing them to Harkonnen aggression anyway, while at the same time falling further and further behind on spice mining as both territory and manpower were reduced. There seemed to be no way out. What were we doing wrong?

As it turned out, a few things.

Sometimes we'd run out of spice to mine, despite knowing that there was more spice to the north, but no longer having access to that area later in the game once the Harkonnens began to advance. Sometimes we'd discover weapons that we could give to the Fremen when training them for combat, but our focus on mining and exploration meant that these weapons wouldn't be put to use until the Harkonnen advance began, by which time it was too late anyway.

With repeated attempts at the game, we eventually realised that the Emperor's ever-increasing demand for spice was not actually related to the size of the spice stockpiles that we were trying to accumulate, but instead seemed to be a slightly randomised number that gradually increased of its own accord. The Emperor's actions in fact functioned as a surrogate time limit mechanism for the game that could not be altered, so our tactic of effectively trying to buy time by mining as much spice as possible was futile. We only ever needed to be mining just enough spice at any time, to keep up with his requests.

We then also realised that the Harkonnens would always begin to attack us after about the same amount of time had passed in the game, regardless of how we had played the game to that point. This solved the riddle of how — or more specifically, when — to mine the spice in the border zone between Atreides and Harkonnen territory: do it as early as possible, before the Harkonnens start to move.

With the understanding that we didn't need to be mining so much all the time after all, that in turn led to a solution to the combat issue. As we'd discover a new cache of weapons somewhere on the map, they'd be given to some of the Fremen tribes that were now free to be trained in combat from the start of the game. They became much more effective fighters with the combination of training for longer and with the earlier supply of weapons.

From then on, everything seemed to more or less fall into place. Once the spice along our northern perimeter had been mined, we'd develop and maintain a line of defensive Fremen forces in that same border area, allowing our mining and prospecting tribes to continue their work in the safer Atreides regions further south. The combat Fremen would fight a war of attrition against the Harkonnen troops, slowly winning more and more territory for the Atreides before culminating in a final battle for the Harkonnen palace itself, where only the largest, most experienced and best equipped Fremen tribes would be capable of victory.

Much like *Begin*, *Dune* was a lesson in making best use of available resources. But within that, the specific lesson learned from *Dune* was that time itself is a resource in its own right. Just because things seem to be going well on the surface for a while, doesn't mean that your mistakes won't start to catch up with you sooner or later.

* * *

One year around 1995, my uncle gave me a book for my birthday called *Making Money Made Simple*.[6] In it, the authors described the power of compound interest: a 16% annual return on investment over 20 years, for example, will return considerably more than the double amount that an 8% return over that same time period would suggest at face value. And the longer you save, the greater that difference. Start saving early, kids!

The same principle applies to gaming as well as to finance. Attentive gamers will look for abilities and bonuses for their characters whose effects will synergise with each other, producing a compounding effect that together adds up to a greater benefit than any two other abilities, which might still be individually beneficial but don't necessarily complement each other.

Take *Twisted Metal 2: World Tour*, for example,[7] which my brother and I regularly hired from the local video store many times before we eventually bought a copy of our own for the original PlayStation console around 1999.

Twisted Metal 2 was a fast-paced action game of car combat, where players choose from a range of different vehicles with different abilities, and that vehicle is then placed into an elimination tournament against other computer-controlled vehicles with abilities of their own, the aim being to simply survive, to be the driver of the last car standing.

As I learned to play the game, my favourite character to play was called Warthog, a sluggish Humvee with average weapons ability, but its good armour allowed me to take a few hits along the way. This seemed easier to get the hang of at first than the fast but weak dune buggy Grasshopper, for example.

Over time, however, I graduated towards the hot pink low rider called Thumper. Reasonably agile although its speed and armour were average, but its special attack was the most powerful in the game: a gigantic flamethrower mounted to the front of the car. Two full blasts of this were enough to completely destroy almost any opponent. But the challenge was in making sure that I could always land the full hit.

In addition to a special attack that was unique to each character, all characters also had access to other abilities like a temporary force field, a jumping ability and the ability to shoot a blast of ice that would momentarily freeze the first opponent that it would strike. That last ability proved particularly synergistic for Thumper: by icing my opponent before unleashing my flamethrower special, I could ensure that I always got the maximum value out of that attack.

Another popular example in my household in the early 2000s was *Diablo II*,[8] a hack-and-slash dungeon crawler game played from an overhead isometric point of view, whose procedurally generated levels ensured that the game's fun was only matched by its replayability. Still always preferring to play the 'good guy' where possible, my character class of choice was the Paladin, a pious warrior type.

Among its many item types, *Diablo II* featured a series of 'set' items. These were collections of three or more pieces of armour that conferred additional bonuses for each additional piece of that armour set that your character wore. While most of these sets were objectively underpowered compared to the best individual items of armour that were also available, many sets remained a perfectly valid option at lower difficulty levels.

But the real demonstration of compounding abilities lay with the paladin's unique lines of combat skills and 'auras', passive abilities that provided further bonuses to the character in addition to the bonuses applied through gear. A paladin could apply a maximum of two such abilities at once, but could switch combinations at any time.

In the early stages of the game, one skill that I favoured was called Zeal, which allowed a paladin to perform additional swings of their weapon per individual attack. My aura of choice was called Thorns, which dealt damage back to any enemy that struck me. Both seemed like reasonable individual choices at the time, but there was no real synergy between them whatsoever.

As I came to understand that the Thorns aura provided more of a defensive benefit than an offensive one like Zeal was, I soon decided to replace Thorns with another aura called Fanaticism. This aura sped up the paladin's attacks, which seemed to combine quite nicely with Zeal; between the two, my character appeared to attack anything and everything around him, almost to the point of his attack action becoming a blur.

The Zeal/Fanaticism combination would see me through the game easily enough on the Normal difficulty setting, and while Nightmare difficulty was more challenging as enemies now came with increased damage resistances, I was able to get through at that setting eventually as well. But the hardest difficulty — Hell — lived up to its name. Many enemies weren't just resistant to various forms of damage, now they were outright immune to some damage types altogether. Under these circumstances, it no longer mattered how fast my attacks were. Something had to change.

Upon further examination of the various options in the skill trees, I picked up another possible combination that might serve me well. Vengeance was a combat skill that added various forms of elemental damage, ensuring that I would at least do some damage with each attack even if enemies were going to be partly immune. My attacks might be slower than with Zeal, but each hit would deal a greater variety of damage types.

Meanwhile, Conviction was an aura that lowered enemy resistances. I'd largely ignored this aura in the earlier stages of the game as most enemies tended not to come with much damage resistance at first anyway. But I soon recognised the value of this aura in partly offsetting one of the key aspects of the harder difficulty levels. And, of course, this effect synergised perfectly with the Vengeance skill.

Now with the Vengeance/Conviction combination, I was able to deal meaningful amounts of damage again, even on Hell difficulty. Over a few years on and off, I managed to play my way through the game one last time, and finally completed it with my paladin having reached level 93 along the way. Considering that every character's death on Hell difficulty also meant that character losing a fair chunk of experience, this represented a pretty decent accomplishment in the end, I thought.

The moral of this story? The total benefits provided by the best combinations of factors can add up to more than the sum of their parts alone.

* * *

The setting and mechanics of some games can give rise to some unexpected behaviour on the part of its players, where certain tactics — while unplanned and possibly unintended on the part of the game's developers — actually take hold as viable and popular styles of play. Nowhere in gaming is this concept of emergent gameplay perhaps more prevalent than in massively multiplayer online games, or MMOs for short.

One of the MMOs I played from 2008 to about 2012 was called *Guild Wars*.[9] This was a fantasy role-playing game with a range of character classes and abilities to choose from, which — unlike most of its contemporaries of the time — did not require a monthly subscription to play, an important factor for any budget-conscious gamer.

Like *Twisted Metal 2* and *Diablo II* before, it became readily apparent in *Guild Wars* that certain combinations of skills and spells were uniquely suited to particular situations, and that much of the search for success in this game relied on learning what worked best, where and when.

My favourite part of *Guild Wars* was the competitive map called Fort Aspenwood, where two opposing teams of eight fought for overall control of a structure on the map within a time limit. One team began with control and would defend against the team of attackers. I personally enjoyed playing both sides over the years, preferring a disruptive mesmer spellcaster when attacking, and a supportive monk healer when defending.

However, I did occasionally catch some unusual behaviour on the part of one or two players on the defending team. Defenders could open and close gates at will while attackers typically had to fight their way through to gain the access that they sought. But every now and then, a defender would deliberately open a gate to allow attackers to advance more easily into the structure. These people were essentially playing for the opposite team and could give the attackers a distinct advantage. Of course, such players were quickly reviled by their own teammates, but the rules of the game allowed for the scenario nonetheless, even if they weren't necessarily intended to.

The game's sequel *Guild Wars 2*,[10] which I played regularly for a few years starting with the beta in 2012, was another game that saw some interesting player tactics emerge, some of which I adopted for myself. As with its predecessor, this was another fantasy MMO set in the same in-game world, but played with an entirely different, more action-oriented feel, as players now had the ability to perform movements like jumping, dodging and swimming.

My favourite mode of play in *Guild Wars 2* was World versus World (WvW), in which three entire servers of players competed across four different maps in week-long matchups for territory and kills; a bit like the Fort Aspenwood of old, except that the maps were far bigger here, with multiple structures of various sizes to battle over all at once.

With the lack of a dedicated healing character class in *Guild Wars 2*, I tended to fall back to my other class of choice from the original game for competitive play: the mesmer. Mesmers provided a unique brand of utility to the game through their powers of denial and confusion; they literally mesmerise unwary opponents with some of the abilities that they possess.

One such ability was a two-part spell called Portal. The mesmer would place one portal on the ground, then had up to 60 seconds to lay a second portal somewhere else nearby. Once both ends of the portal were lit, as many as 20 allied players could teleport themselves through the portal from one end to the other before it closed.

I used to apply portals quite a lot to provide shortcuts to incoming friendly forces during defensive combat situations. I'd be one of a handful of players holed up inside a tower that was under siege by a larger attacking force; the first portal would be laid inside the tower, then I'd run out towards our reinforcements and light up the other end to let them all directly inside. These 'portcuts' often came as a surprise to the enemy, who might otherwise have expected an easier fight inside the tower than what they actually got. Many a structure was saved over the years with this tactic.

Sometimes, though, reinforcements were in short supply, and that would mean having no choice but to surrender the structure to the invaders. But for a lone mesmer, the battle didn't necessarily have to end there. Keeps, in particular, were large enough for someone to hide away in certain corners that, if not checked by the invaders post-capture, would allow a mesmer to simply wait for their enemies to disperse. Then once the coast was clear, they could call in some friends towards their position, lay a portal from the inside of the keep to the outside to let their friends straight back in, and the keep could easily be retaken with a minimum of opposition, without having to spend time and resources breaking down any gates and/or walls first.

Over time, awareness of this mesmer tactic grew and smarter opponents would usually take the time to 'sweep' a keep after it had been captured, so it gradually became more and more difficult to successfully hide away. But mesmers themselves were able to develop a few more tricks to stay ahead of the game for a while.

As well as the range of character classes that a player had to choose from when starting a new character in *Guild Wars* 2, there were also five different playable races available, each of various physical sizes. For a WvW mesmer looking to play hide-and-seek, the best race for this purpose was the gnome-like asura, for their diminutive stature. An oversized norn or charr mesmer, though? Not so much.

However, some mesmers who had happened to choose a race other than asura — myself included — eventually realised that they didn't have to suffer for their inherent size disadvantage. The game also offered a range of potions called tonics, that could change a player's appearance to something completely different. With the right tonic, any mesmer could turn themselves into a creature even smaller than an asura, called a quaggan. Becoming a quaggan allowed mesmers to hide in some places that would otherwise have guaranteed discovery.

But there was one thing even shorter than a quaggan: the portal spell itself. A mesmer could lay a portal, then actually jump outside of the structure and wait there in relative safety for up to a minute before they would have to let themselves back in. This meant that sweepers wouldn't find anybody inside the keep at all, for the first 50 seconds or so of their search. So if their search was sufficiently brief and the portal itself was not found, a mesmer could sometimes avoid detection entirely by hiding outside of the structure rather than inside it, even if the keep had actually been swept.

At my best, I could lay a portal in the right place, wait outside for just under a minute, then light up the other end, turn myself into a quaggan and then teleport back in. At all times it was still possible for me to be found, and at no time was there ever any cheating involved, but it remained a decently effective strategy for as long as I was regularly playing the game. And it made me no shortage of in-game friends along the way, too.

Like many other games of the past, *Guild Wars 2* was all about creative use of available options and discovering which combinations of options provided the best results. But this particular game also served to remind me not to ignore the potential possibilities when combining even the seemingly strangest of bedfellows, to leave no proverbial stone unturned. Only through continual experimentation can one truly claim to have identified the most effective strategies for success.

So, hopefully, one can understand that all those years of nerding out behind a computer screen might not have been the complete waste of time that some might have claimed them to be, after all. For their service as a coping mechanism particularly during the earlier years, and the life lessons they were able to teach me along the way, consciously or otherwise, I have very few regrets about having grown up a gamer.

It almost made up for my being fat throughout that entire time.

Almost.

3 THE FAT GUY

I am confident no man labouring under obesity can be quite insensible to the sneers and remarks of the cruel and injudicious in public assemblies, public vehicles, or the ordinary street traffic. ... I am as regardless of public remark as most men, but I have felt these difficulties and therefore avoided such circumscribed accommodation and notice, and by that means have been deprived of many advantages to health and comfort.
—William Banting, Letter on Corpulence, *1864*[1]

WHEN I WAS GROWING UP, I wanted to be a meteorologist. At this point in my life I find it hard to explain why, but I suppose I was fascinated by the world around me in some weird way, and wanted a career that would indulge that curiosity, while at the same time playing to my relative academic strengths in maths and science. The subject would be relatable in the real world as well; even if we don't really care about it all that much, how often do we all find ourselves talking about the weather anyway?

That soon changed during high school, however, when I explored the sorts of qualifications that would be required for such a career, the details of which escape me now, but essentially would have meant several more years of study at university.

This was a problem. While I did particularly well in some subjects in each of Years 10, 11 and 12, my weakest subjects were getting worse over time. I could feel myself getting sick of school in general. I just wanted to get out into the real world, get a job and live my life. I could always choose to go back to school again later if I wanted.

But what sort of career options were there for people who didn't want to stay in school at that point? And within those options, what would suit a guy who really wanted to live within his physical means, to avoid as much exercise as possible?

My extracurricular activities during high school were few and far between. I was your classic fat ginger nerd, a semi-regular at the library and a very-regular in the computer labs. While I represented the school in regional social studies competitions, spelling bees and the like, they weren't so much dreams of mine as they were cases of me not objecting to taking part when others might have.

But these experiences would all come together when an opportunity arose to join the school's radio club as an occasionally rostered member. Each week different students would record a half-hour programme of high school news and popular music, for broadcast on the town's local radio station on Sunday mornings.

There were enough students involved that each of us only got two or three chances across the year. But it was enough for the bug to bite. Here seemed the ideal career for me: sitting around, pushing buttons, playing music. Sure, there was talking required as well, but I'd never had any fear of public speaking going back to my earlier school days, and in this scenario it was easy to rationalise the idea even further. I would be in a small room by myself, surrounded by equipment; essentially talking to no-one, to nothing but a microphone wrapped in a foam sock.

And so at the start of my last year of high school, when the radio station itself advertised publicly for a part-time announcer to cover weekends, I had no hesitation in applying. When they invited me in for an audition a few weeks later, I was sat in the same recording studio that we'd used for the school programme the previous year, only this time I was by myself. They handed me some written material to read back: a couple of news stories, a couple of ad scripts and a weather forecast. Oh look, I get to talk about the weather.

The end result was apparently good enough, and all of a sudden in March of 1995 at the age of 16 years and 5 months, I became — to my knowledge — the youngest announcer ever employed by New Zealand state-owned radio at that time.

There were lots of things I came to enjoy about that job. The entire show was performed live; every song — whether it was a record, cartridge or CD — was cued and started by me, every sting or ad break was loaded and triggered by me, every phone call made or received on the air was set up by me. The news came beaming in remotely, live at the top of the hour, to the second. I took a great deal of pride in being able to 'time out' each hour so that the content would finish precisely on time for the next news bulletin.

My presentation style was fairly straightforward. I could neither be considered the most charismatic, nor the most comedic, but technically I was generally very accurate. Once I'd gotten the hang of things, there was very little 'dead air', very few mistakes.

But the best thing of all was that nobody got to see me in my work. Unless they knew me personally, the listeners would never really know what I looked like. Of course, what I looked like was something resembling an albino walrus, but that was my little secret that a job like this would allow me to keep from the world. No-one needs to know.

After a few months I decided that this would be the life for me beyond school, but there were no full-time vacancies forthcoming at the station there, so during that year my mother and I negotiated a full-time announcing position with the new privately owned station that had just started up across town. This would start once I had finished that year of high school, but the agreement had been made well in advance, only halfway through the year.

It was a strange position to be in. Everyone else I knew was wondering and worrying about what they were going to do with themselves once high school was over, but I already had a plan worked out six months in advance. The only catch was that I couldn't tell anyone about it, and certainly not my current employer. When one of my full-time colleagues told our boss she was also leaving for the opposition, she was given her marching orders that very day. The real world, it turns out, can be pretty serious business.

I imagine it was stranger still to others, when some of my grades took a complete nosedive halfway through the year. They couldn't know the reason why at the time, but it was simply that with the job already having been arranged no matter my results, I just lost all interest in doing anything any more in any of the subjects that I didn't enjoy.

And that's pretty much the story behind how I came to fail high school English. My marks were okay after six months but, without having any need to pretend to care about Shakespeare any more, I did literally nothing else there for the rest of the year and wound up with 46% at the end.

Still, that was better than my final PE score.

Despite all of the drama that it created along the way, however, the secret itself was successfully kept safe. No more than six people knew the truth behind that year's mixed grades, right through to the end. The final decision to not return to school the following year was confirmed, and I debuted across town as a full-time weekday afternoon announcer in February 1996.

Most of the time I was left to my own devices in the studio, and so for most of that time I was happy to just do my thing, out of sight if not out of mind. There was the occasional outside appearance, for which I had to wear the station's uniform: a bright yellow polo shirt two sizes too small for me. Not the most fetching of fashion statements for most normal-sized people, let alone a fatty like me. Where possible, I would volunteer to be the one controlling the broadcast from the studio instead.

For the next couple of years, I biked to work just as I'd biked to school. Not that it ever seemed to benefit me physically of course; I remained as humungous as always. But it was a long way to have to ride when it rained, and I was becoming an inconvenience in relying on others to ferry me around in bad weather.

In part, I had resisted the idea of getting my driver's licence because I was afraid of what that would do for my weight. After all, my exercise would fall away almost completely if I were to transition from a bicycle to a car. But the pressure mounted and finally I got around to gaining my licence in the autumn of 1998.

My first car was a 1989 Honda Civic. The paintwork was a metallic silver, but on the paperwork it was listed as 'pink', which was always cause for an internal cringe whenever I took it in for a warrant or service. I was a very nervous driver at first, but she and I became more comfortable with each other over time. I soon named her Flattery, since ... you know, she got me everywhere.

However, my growth in confidence was sadly now being matched by further growth to my waistline, just as I'd feared it would. It was slow growth over the following years, but growth it was, nonetheless: 122kg, 123, 124, ...

One of my work colleagues from around this time felt that I needed to embrace my size, and tried to come up with a handle for me that people could use on air. He meant well, I suppose, but I was never comfortable with any of his ideas from the start. 'Big Red?' No. 'The Round Man of Sound?' Even worse. My name on its own would be fine, thank you very much. I didn't need a description to go along with it.

And besides, some listeners apparently already knew me well enough without the need for such a description anyway. One such person phoned in one evening for a song request. 'Can I hear the song *You Sexy Thing*?'

'Sure,' I answered. 'And who's that for?'

'That's for ... Brendan Reid!' came the reply, followed by maniacal laughter before they hung up.

I didn't play their song.

Beyond even the prank calls were the prank gifts. On Valentine's Day one year I received a great big bouquet of flowers at the station, addressed to me from a 'secret admirer'. That one really hurt. My colleagues tried to make light of it, but I immediately called bullshit. If anybody were truly serious about that sort of thing with me, they only needed to say so in person. In a job where one was required to put on a happy face all day every day, that particular day was tough.

The wider I grew, the more desperately I tried to hide it all away. I even fashioned for myself a horrible neckbeard somewhere around 1999, in a pitiful attempt to disguise my extra chin, that otherwise seemed to transition directly into my swollen neck. Jawline, what jawline? I made a promise to myself at that time, that for as long as I was unhappy with how I looked, I would never go clean-shaven again.

By the turn of the millennium I had been promoted to the breakfast show. Professionally it felt like a natural progression, but on a personal level it was something that I tired of fairly quickly. Literally, of course, having to get up so much earlier in the mornings now than ever before, but figuratively as well. Being the primetime anchor meant a higher community profile for me, and there were more commercial obligations to be met accordingly. More public appearances, more broadcasts on location, more out and about.

This was not what I'd originally gotten into the business for. People were now beginning to recognise me on the street. Most of them were nice enough to my face, but given my history, it was easy to imagine them all thinking very differently behind my back. My younger brother, still in high school at this stage, mentioned to me once that a girl had told him I 'sounded hot'. He didn't have to work hard to disappoint her when he told her the truth.

One of the more memorable public appearances that I put in one summer was when I took part in a game of cricket at the local oval, with a mish-mash of local 'celebrities' taking on what more or less amounted to a shadow regional representative team, all for charity. Many were surprised when I put my hand up for this, myself included. I assumed there would be various unpleasantries that I'd have to deal with, but, on the other hand, it was possibly the only chance I'd ever have at playing a real, actual game of cricket, with proper gear and everything. Fat people can have dreams, too.

The first of those unpleasantries was handed to me a day or two before the game: a beige-coloured T-shirt that was to serve as our team's uniform. It was described to me as 'one size fits all', yet was even smaller than the station's own bright yellow polo shirt. I debated long and hard over which would be less embarrassing: to wear something comfortable of my own, or stretch the hell out of what was given to me, and just suck in my gut as best I could. The latter option won out in the end; better to be mocked for being fat, than to be mocked for being both fat and selfish.

On the morning itself, I set my goals deliberately low; I knew I was seriously out of my depth here as far as my playing ability was concerned. If I could at least score a run, I'd be happy. If I got a chance to bowl, a wicket would be an absolute dream. Especially in front of the family, some of whom would also be there watching.

I don't remember who won the toss, but we fielded first. I wanted a fielding position closer than where I was placed on the boundary, since I wasn't really up for running, or throwing, or as it would turn out, catching. One ball went sky high in my direction and I managed to carefully watch it all the way into my hands. Except that to unfamiliar hands, catching a real cricket ball feels an awful lot like catching a rock. The pain of the impact came as a shock, the ball popped right back out again before I could clasp it, and down it went. There was no hiding me in the best of moments let alone that one, no matter how much I wanted the ground to just swallow me up then and there.

The other side, being full of guys who actually knew how to play, were racking up the runs fairly comfortably, so most of us were given a shot with the ball just to mix things up a bit. Still, it was a nice surprise to be waved over to the northern end when I was, especially considering what had just happened in the outfield.

I took a moment behind the crease for a bit of perspective. The pitch was far longer than I was used to on the neighbour's tennis court. The leggies would be best put away in favour of more straightforward off-breaks that I could control better, especially in that grossly undersized T-shirt, where producing any sort of proper bowling action was always going to be a challenge.

The first over went well enough; I think I only got whacked for a couple of boundaries. But it ended even better when the final delivery was skied once again in the direction where I'd been fielding earlier. This time, though, the fielder out there made no mistake, and I officially had a wicket to my name.

A drinks break immediately followed, and I presumed that would be all for the struggling fat guy. But no, I was asked to ~~attempt to~~ roll the arm over some more on the other side of the break as well. Maybe it was the wicket that earned me a reprieve? I don't know.

I overstepped a few times in the second over, but there were no markers around that I knew of for me to properly mark my run-up. Was I supposed to have brought my own? I was told that all gear would be provided? Never mind.

By my third over, I felt I was starting to get the hang of things and began mixing up the deliveries just a little. One straighter ball rapped the batsman's pads low and in front, and although he had taken some stride forward, I instinctively turned and gave a long, loud appeal to the umpire. To my delight, he raised his finger and I had wicket number two! Fist pump!

That joy didn't last long, however. The next guy in knew exactly what he was doing when he immediately carted me for three straight sixes back over my head, bringing an inevitable end to my bowling spell. My figures were 2 for 42 ... off three overs.

I remember gearing up in the tent while waiting for my turn to bat, somewhat worried for my safety for when my turn would come. Still, the opposition bowlers were at least being limited to a run-up of just a few paces, and being wrapped up in all that padding made me feel a little more secure.

The wickets fell steadily to no-one's surprise, and before long it was my turn to head out there at about number 8 or so in the batting order. I had asked not to be put right at the tail in the hope that I would get enough of an opportunity to score something, anything. They granted me that much, at least.

The first few deliveries were full, but outside the off stump. I was too afraid to try to come forward for the drive, preferring to wait for a shorter one at that width. Suddenly it came, a wild attempt at a cut shot actually connected, and the ball raced away to the third man region for a single. I was so proud of myself that I was tempted to raise my bat at the other end as if I'd scored a hundred, but I refrained. I wasn't popular enough to get away with making any more of a fool of myself than I was already doing.

I lost a couple of partners while I was out there, and to my astonishment I found myself briefly playing the senior partner. But that wasn't to last; the bowlers had worked out that I wasn't too keen on coming forward to the ball, and one straight yorker was all it took to rattle the stumps, after having collected my way to five runs.

The game ended soon after, and we'd been predictably hammered. But with plenty of time to spare, both sides agreed that my team would now be given a second innings to bat.

If only they'd told me that *before* I'd filled up on soft drink, having believed my day was over at that point, and not after.

Going out there a second time I was not feeling at all well, and the opposition picked up on it too. Some of the close-in fielders began loudly exchanging fat jokes. Really, guys? Was it not enough to have already won the day so comfortably against a bunch of amateurs? I guess not. I edged one delivery through the slip cordon for a couple of runs. It might have been worth three had my belly not been swimming as it was, but at least it shut them up for a few moments while they had to go fetch.

The following over I was clean bowled once again, and finally the day was truly done.

So my scores were five runs and then two. I'd contributed to the occasion, and my feeble little goals had been more than met. I should have felt happy, but I wasn't. I couldn't ignore the fact that across the day, nobody had really acknowledged me more than they absolutely had to.

Nobody had welcomed me into the team that morning, but they were all happy enough to meet each other. There were no high-fives or pats on the back for either of my wickets, but the catching fielder collected plenty of both. And the T-shirt more than did its part to hinder me physically.

But it was the sledging at the end that made it undeniably clear: I did not belong out there that day, nor would I ever belong out there on any other day. Everybody believed it, by the end even me.

I might have ticked one off for the bucket list, but my love for the game was permanently damaged as a consequence. I don't think I even played in the backyard any more after that.

* * *

One of the best things about leaving home and moving into my own place was that I finally had a phone line all to myself. We had the internet at my parents' place for a couple of years before I moved out, but in a household of six, there was always competition for access to the phone. Hardly a day went by when I wasn't yelled at for tying up the line.

I'd had a few flatmates on and off during those early years to help split the bills, but I didn't mind living alone either. Those were the times when I always felt safest to go searching online for that forbidden topic, that no-one was allowed to know that I was constantly thinking about: how to lose weight.

Eating less hadn't worked. Neither did moving more really, although moving less had contributed to further gain when Flattery came along. So how had other people done it?

According to the internet, most people were apparently finding success doing just what I'd tried and failed to do. Eat less, move more. Calories in, calories out. This was maddening. What the hell was wrong with me for that approach not to have worked for me too?

It still doesn't make any sense. It's not fair.

A few people were talking about another kind of diet called the Atkins diet. It was being spoken of like it was some revolutionary game-changing deal, where people would drop dozens of pounds in a matter of weeks. Well, that just sounded too good to be true. And it certainly didn't gel at all with the official dietary advice that I was already well familiar with. It had to be a scam.

Still, at one point around 2002 I remember it actually making the news on TV. This Atkins thing was all the rage in the States, apparently. Eat bacon and eggs, they said. Eat steak and butter, they said. Well, mainstream media would have none of that. Out came all the usual responses, decrying Atkins as a ridiculous, even dangerous 'fad' diet. All that fat will clog your arteries and give you a heart attack! And, of course, I listened. These were the experts in their field, after all. So that was officially scratched.

The next idea I picked up from somewhere was to buy an ab roller. You know, one of those little wheeled things with two handles on them, where you roll forward on your knees and the internal spring-loaded mechanism helps you back up to your knees again? Those things that are small enough to pack away at the back of your wardrobe, so no-one ever knows that you even own one? Yeah, I owned one.

This was an attempt to target the very worst part of me: my stomach. If I could at least improve that to some extent, then maybe I wouldn't look so physically out of proportion.

To its credit, I could certainly feel it whenever I tried it. But the problem was that the wheel would either leave a long indent in the carpet, collecting fluff as it went, or it would leave a long mark on the kitchen vinyl. Either way, this was evidence to others that I had been trying something, which I just couldn't bear to leave behind under any circumstances.

I didn't think to place a mat of some kind on top of the surface I was rolling on. To be fair, when I think back now, I would probably have had to buy such a mat anyway, which itself would also have been a dead giveaway. But as a result, that ab roller instead spent most of the next few years collecting dust at the back of the wardrobe.

By 2003 the neckbeard had been reduced to a slightly less embarrassing goatee. I had moved to Christchurch having retired from the radio, and was now pursuing a career in IT. I was fortunate to live in a flat just a few blocks from where I was studying. I had hoped that with a return to at least some physical activity again as I was now walking to and from classes, maybe the weight situation might improve?

Nope: 126kg, 127, 128, ...

I figured that my diet probably wasn't great, even if I wasn't really sure what to do about it. There was only fast food once on weekends, but amongst the odd fruit and veges were lots of chuck-whatever-into-the-microwave during the week. Pizzas, pies, noodles and, above all, sandwiches. Lots and lots of sandwiches. Well, some of these things might have had a bit of fat in them, but all that cutting fat had ever done for me was make me hungry, so what else was I supposed to do?

While studying I had a part-time job, working as a store person for a retail chain. They had a strict uniform policy, requiring black dress shoes for all employees, even though this particular employee was almost never seen by customers, and such footwear wasn't all that practical in a back dock type environment anyway. Never mind that dress shoes aren't all that comfortable for fatties in pretty much any other environment either. In the end I would ride the line by wearing my own sneakers most days, but kept the dress shoes on hand for whenever regional managers or higher would visit.

Post-study, I started a new full-time IT job in the city at the end of 2006; this meant a slightly longer walk to work than it had been to class, but not by much. Still, I really tried to make something of this evolution in my routine; I would walk to and from work in casual clothing so that I could really power through it, and then change to proper work gear on site. Perhaps if I tried really hard, it might just be enough to turn the tide?

Nope: 129kg, 130, 131, ...

Clothes shopping was steadily becoming more and more difficult. There weren't many places that sold 4XL shirts, let alone 5XL ones. Every time I found one in either size I would buy it then and there, and just hope that it would somehow fit me when I got home. Pants were even harder to find, and most of the time I had to get the legs reduced in length because I needed the waist so wide. My wardrobe was accumulating with clothes that were too small for me, in the forlorn hope that one day I might be able to fit some of them again.

I hated my picture being taken, for obvious reasons. For many years I was successful in avoiding most situations where I might have expected to be photographed. However, one shot slipped onto social media in 2007 when a friend posted a picture of me stalking a dalek at a local comic book convention. That had otherwise been a really enjoyable weekend, with some great celebrity panels, lots of toys and comics on display and even a local wrestling show. But having not seen myself from the outside in some time, I was so mortified at my appearance in this photo that I immediately untagged my name from it, and hid it from my timeline.

While on the way home from work one day, I caught a conversation on the radio between the hosts who were joking to each other about fat people, wondering aloud why others don't just 'give them a chance?' One woman rang in and was pretty straightforward about it. 'When I see a fat guy,' she explained, 'I see someone who doesn't know how to take care of themselves. And if they don't know how to take care of themselves, how could they possibly take care of anyone else? How could they possibly take care of a family?' Her argument made immediate, perfect and depressing sense. My high school prediction was well on track: I would die alone and before my time.

And all the while, the weight creep continued: 132kg, 133, 134, …

One evening in 2009 I began to feel an odd sensation in my chest. It wasn't so much pain, but just a general sort of discomfort in the area, like my chest was somehow just trying to remind me that it was there. I was pretty tired that night anyway, so I figured I'd just sleep it off, and I'd be right again in the morning.

But then I noticed when I lay down that the odd sensation was definitely becoming more painful. I sat up again and it eased, I lay back down and it got worse again.

Sleep had long been one of my favourite things in life. After all, for as long as I was sleeping, I couldn't possibly be eating and therefore sleep couldn't possibly make me any fatter. But if this feeling in my chest was going to prevent me from getting some quality shut-eye, then I needed to do something about it. So I called the local toll-free Healthline service and described my symptoms. They immediately referred me to an ambulance, which took me away to hospital that very evening.

I spent the night in the emergency department there while they ran some tests. But they couldn't really find much wrong with me at first. My electrocardiogram was showing mostly the right sort of noise, my blood pressure was normal, my chest X-ray came out clear. Some ibuprofen dealt with the immediate pain issue, so I was finally able to get some sleep.

The following day I was transferred to a ward while they waited for the outcome of a few more tests. My blood sugar was slightly elevated but not excessively. The same was true of my cholesterol. The doctor was definitely surprised to see that; he told me that had cholesterol standards not recently been tightened, my total number would have been considered completely normal. Aside from being really fat, there didn't appear to be much wrong with me at all.

In the end they decided that while they weren't sure exactly what to diagnose, their best guess was pericarditis, inflammation of the area that surrounds the heart, but not of the heart itself. Apparently this was something that could just happen to anybody, and I should just take more ibuprofen for the pain, should it ever return. Oh, and my potassium levels were also a bit low. 'What foods are high in potassium?' I asked. Their answers were bananas and chocolate. No problem, I didn't mind either of those.

By 2010 I had reached 135kg. One day in May of that year, after beginning to hear more and more in the news about how particularly unhealthy sugary soft drinks were, I decided to try a little experiment and replaced all soft drinks with water. At the same time I also bought a fan bike; think an exercycle, but with arms that also oscillated in time with the pedals. I hadn't ridden a bike since before I'd gotten my driver's licence, but I was both too self-conscious and too scared to go riding around outside in the big city where I lived now.

A strange thing began to happen at that point. I say it was strange because it had never happened to me before, and given my sorry track record to date, I had no reason to expect that it would start happening now. But for the first time in my life, the scales began to slowly work their way backwards. Over the following four months I managed to lose a total of 7kg. I couldn't believe my eyes. This was incredibly exciting!

I presumed that the primary reason for this was not the exercise, because I'd never been able to lose any weight from any other exercise before. So it had to be the sugar. But things got confusing pretty quickly when I went looking for other sources of sugar to cut out from my diet. For example, there was sugar in fruit juice, but that comes from fruit so that has to be good for me, right? And I was still trying to stay mindful of following the healthy food pyramid where possible, still eating lots of bread and potatoes, because that's what a good boy would do.

Before I could think it all through any further, however, things would soon take another surprise turn. Early one Saturday morning in September 2010, I was woken by what felt like a small-to-moderately sized earthquake. Such tremors are not uncommon in New Zealand, but that doesn't make each experience any less unpleasant.

I sat up in bed for a few moments waiting for it to stop, but instead the movement suddenly took off to a whole new level that I'd never felt before. I instinctively leapt towards the bedroom doorway and held on while the world around me was shunted in an unnaturally exaggerated left-right rhythm, over and over. And what a noise it made in the night: there came the sounds of smaller things falling down inside, larger things like chimneys and brick fences falling down outside, and a thunderous rumbling that roared up from the ground itself.

This powerful temblor marked the beginning of an especially difficult personal period for me. As scary as the event itself was, I could still rationalise it as only having lasted for no more than a minute before settling down again. It should have been easy to just compartmentalise the whole experience and file it away under 'life'.

Except it wasn't. For weeks on end, the city was bombarded with regular aftershocks at all hours of every day and night, each one triggering a fresh reminder of the original. The first one had started small, so every new small one had the potential to become another new big one.

The weight loss stalled. Perhaps this was as much from the stress of the situation as anything else? I wasn't sure. I certainly found it impossible to relax, living every moment constantly on edge, always worried about 'the next one'. I began to develop a habit of having the TV on in the house at all times during the day, so that I wouldn't be set off so easily by the likes of a truck rumbling down the road outside, or even the occasional gust of wind.

At night, not only did the radio have to stay on, but so did the light beside my bed. The big one had happened at night, after all; I needed to be ready at literally any moment. But I needed my sleep too, and that was becoming so difficult that I would drive myself out of town every Friday night to spend the weekends with my parents, just so I could get at least two good nights of sleep a week. During the week, I began to rely on half a zopiclone pill each night to knock me out.

The aftershocks seemed to have eased somewhat by Christmas, but another sharp jolt centred right under the city on Boxing Day saw me spend much of the New Year's holidays out of town again. I began to consider leaving the city altogether, and booked a few sessions with a counsellor to make sure that I was looking at things from a complete perspective. 'I could tell you that there will be another aftershock,' I remember saying to him, 'and I will only ever be wrong once.'

He encouraged me not to feel guilty about my situation, and to go ahead with finding the sense of control that I was clearly missing. Essentially it came down to a choice of fight or flight, and I felt that there was never a chance of winning any fight against such forces of nature.

So I decided to pursue plans to move away. I started looking around online for job prospects elsewhere in the country in January 2011, and by February I had begun offloading possessions from the flat, so that I would have less to move once I had actually found something somewhere else.

But later that February, my time ran out. It was a Tuesday afternoon at about ten to one. I was writing an email at work, my mind drifting ahead in anticipation of a chicken and mushroom fettuccine from the pasta place downstairs for lunch. Mmm, sweet nourishing pasta ...

My daydream was rudely interrupted when all of a sudden the entire building gave a single massive lurch, as if a runaway army tank had just crashed into it from the street. 'Whoa!' I exclaimed, instinctively sliding my chair away from the desk, hands raised. My three colleagues in the office at the time were similarly surprised.

A short pause followed, then the building suddenly began heaving again, only this time it didn't stop. I was thrown from the chair to my knees as everything around me turned to complete chaos. The doorway was only a couple of metres away, but the desk was closer still, so I scrambled underneath it and curled up into a huddle. I made peace with myself then and there. When they pick through the rubble, at least they'll find me in the right place.

I could feel the floor beneath my legs twisting and contorting, every violent new movement taking its own unique direction. There was no rhythm to it at all this time. Up, down, left, right, punch, kick, again, again and again.

The power went out, the office now bathed in shadow. I glanced up to see the computer case being shunted towards the front edge of the desk. Do I try to stop it and risk my hand, or do I let it fall and lose my work? I reached out and gave it a quick shove back towards its proper place.

From then on, all I could do in the half-darkness was just crouch, hold, wait and listen. If the ground was giving out a rumble this time I couldn't hear it, but there were plenty of other noises to take in. The building itself was groaning with each convulsion. I could hear ceiling tiles dancing in their cavities, glass smashing, larger objects like filing cabinets and shelving occasionally crashing over, smaller objects flying about like ice cubes flung from an open blender.

And above it all was the screaming. But these weren't the light-hearted sorts of squeals that people might make while watching a horror movie. These screams came from people who were putting their entire bodies into the expression, as if it were to be the last sound they would ever make. They came from people who truly believed, in that moment, that they were going to die.

Finally, just as reality itself seemed ready to come down all around us ... it didn't. The shaking stopped, and the noises were reduced to a few crying voices, and the occasional rustling of scattered paperwork as it settled wherever it would. A discordant hum of building and car alarms now filled the background from the outside, a soundtrack as twisted as the newfound nature of my very surroundings.

I heard my colleagues calling out to each other. 'Oh my God, are you all right?' It sounded like everybody else was okay, until they realised someone was missing. 'Wait, where's Brendan?'

They found me still crouched, silent and unmoving beneath my desk, seemingly unharmed but still paralysed with fear.

Many people died that day. Many more were injured, myself included. I sprained ligaments in my knee which made walking difficult for several weeks, and while it's possible that it happened when the quake began, I'll never know for sure as I didn't actually notice any physical discomfort until later that evening. Presumably I was just running on so much adrenalin at the time.

Mentally, though, I was completely broken and I immediately knew it. The aftershock sequence had effectively been reset back to the beginning, and I knew that I wasn't going to be able to cope with another five months like the last five had been. For the first time I felt like I had an even bigger problem than being fat. Now I had to work out how I was just going to live.

I wandered home in a dusty daze, having decided on the way back that I was going to leave town that night. At first I was relieved to see that the flat itself was still standing when I arrived, though I was freshly shocked to discover that the carport had collapsed, an overhead beam having crushed the roof and windscreen of my dear Flattery. She wouldn't be getting me anywhere further any more.

But I was still determined to make it out that night, and make it out I did, dodgy knee and all. I packed a bag of clothes, and managed to hitch three different rides from my central city flat, all the way out to Mum's place. Finding each ride was actually easier than it might have been on any other day; it wasn't like there was any shortage of traffic leaving the city that afternoon.

I'm not sure if it'll ever be possible for me to put the events of that day completely behind me. I know I'm still not there yet. As much as I didn't want to at the time, I returned once the following week with a moving van to recover what household contents hadn't been shattered by it all, and a couple more times for work meetings for a day each. But it would be a full nine years before I would find the courage to spend just a single night in Christchurch again.

4 THE MOMENT

People encounter impasses on simple problems that they are competent to solve because the presentation of the problem triggers the retrieval or activation of prior knowledge that blocks the solution. Changes in the inappropriate initial representation allow previously unheeded possibilities to come to mind; this is the moment of insight.

—*Günther Knoblich, Stellan Ohlsson and Gary E. Raney,* An eye movement study of insight problem solving, *2001*[1]

EXACTLY ONE MONTH to the day following the February 2011 earthquake, I moved into a new flat down the road in Timaru, where the company I was working for had also chosen to relocate. I'd already found a new car down there, and given how many other people there were who also had the same idea as me, to just get the hell out of Christchurch after what had happened, I considered myself very lucky to have acquired both.

I wanted to help with the move more than I was able to, but my sprained knee prevented me from doing any heavy lifting, so most of that work was left to the guys from the moving company instead. I did what I could around them anyway of course, and they were fine to deal with face to face of course, but it was easy to imagine that they thought I was faking an injury, and I was just being lazy because I was fat. Of course.

The town was a very comfortable fit at first. It didn't have any high standards to live up to or anything, it just had to be free of shaking. This alone was an immediate relief. I also quickly appreciated that after having spent almost my entire life on the plains, this was the first place I'd ever lived in that came with a view. It was an upstairs unit near the top of a hill. I could see all the way to the Southern Alps on a clear day, with the suburbs in the foreground and, from one window, even a little bit of the sea.

Still, the plan was never to stay there too long, just enough to take stock, reboot my life and make some new plans. Going through my things, I soon realised that I'd somehow lost my stash of zopiclone during the move. Going cold turkey made those first few nights there a little nervy, but without the constant aftershocks to have to deal with any more, I was soon able to manage again.

My weight had rebounded slightly, but stabilised at about 130kg. My fan bike was still in one piece, and was actually proving quite a useful rehabilitation tool for my injured knee. Both my TV and microwave had been smashed and needed to be replaced, and my computer was acting a bit flaky and needed repairs, but I still had my old bed, my fridge, washing machine and recliner.

I also still had most of my clothes, and, having hurriedly thrown them all into large plastic rubbish bags for the move south, the process of unpacking them again now made me realise just how much of my wardrobe was hopelessly too small for me by this point. Even with my modest weight loss of the previous year, I was still a monster. I'm still going to be fat forever, and there's still nothing I can do about it.

So I took that opportunity to have a good wardrobe clear-out. A lot of stuff was clothing-binned that day, though not quite everything. Of the things that clearly didn't fit me any more, only a few items of special historical note made the cut, like that bright yellow polo shirt from my earlier radio days, for example. Even if it was about four sizes too small for me now. Hmph.

For the next few months I tried to settle into a new daily routine, which was much the same as the old one: the same work with the same people but just in a different environment, with different lunch options. There was a bakery down the road on one side and a noodle house on the other, and a fast food outlet in the opposite direction. I also found a really nice Indian restaurant that made these amazing cheesy naan breads. Sooo good.

I wasn't sure if I could feel myself getting any better mentally with time, but all along I believed I was better off there than I would have been back up the road in Christchurch. This feeling was reinforced in no uncertain terms when another large aftershock rocked the city in June, which even down in Timaru still felt big enough to cause a good scare.

One day in October I heard the local radio station advertising a vacancy for a part-time announcer. It had been a while for me for sure, but maybe this would be just the ticket to help boost my flagging confidence. The station was more than happy to take on someone with my experience, and I soon settled into an occasional Saturday afternoon role around my other full-time work that I was still doing during the week.

Towards the end of 2011 my weekday work colleagues made the collective decision to return to Christchurch. They felt like it was time, though I strongly disagreed. Had they insisted on my going back with them, I was fully prepared to walk away and push for more hours at the radio station instead. However they took my concerns seriously, and instead arranged for me to continue to work remotely from Timaru, by myself in a small windowless room at the back of the building next door to the one we were all leaving.

This I thought would be manageable, and it was for at least a short while. But for the first time in my life, I soon began to experience a surprising sense of loneliness.

As a natural introvert, I tire easily when spending extended periods of time with large enough groups of people, and have always been more comfortable by myself, given the choice. At this point in my life I was well used to living in solitude which was fine, and working alone might have been fine as well if I'd had company to come home to, but being alone at all hours of the day at once was feeling like just a little too much. Often the only time I would have any reason to talk to anybody at all on any given day was when I went out to order lunch. Even the occasional weekend radio shift didn't seem to be helping, perhaps because most of the conversation I was having there was still one-way.

This loneliness, coupled with the still-lingering fear of the next big aftershock, led me to seek out further counselling. I've never been afraid of counsellors, and have never been afraid to admit that every now and then when things get bad enough, I feel like I might need the services of one. Like in Christchurch a year earlier, this to me was just another one of those times.

We worked through my recent history, and while she wasn't qualified to formally diagnose me with post-traumatic stress disorder, she felt that, in her own words, I was 'exhibiting some of the symptoms.' We agreed that I needed to sort my life out and find a new job, working with a team of people again, and preferably in a bigger town that was likely to offer a few more future career options.

My first choice was Dunedin. I'd always had a soft spot for the south, having been born in the region and still having extended family links in the area, including an aunt and uncle in the city itself. The cost of living wasn't too bad compared to many other parts of the country. And the weather was a little cooler as well, which was important for a fatty like me. Summers had always felt too hot for as long as I could remember. Unlike most other people, there was always a limit to how many layers that I could personally peel off, before those around me might start to get a bit upset about it.

I applied for a couple of new positions directly, before catching the attention of a recruiting agency who soon began to feed me some additional opportunities. After a few months I was able to secure another IT position in the city, but with the catch that they wanted me to start down there as soon as possible.

So I waved goodbye to both of my Timaru jobs in late 2012, and spent a frantic few weeks trying to find a place to live further south before my new job there began. I wanted somewhere small, but hopefully within walking distance of the central city so I could at least maintain that amount's worth of regular exercise.

With time running out, I settled on a nice small place — halfway up another hill — that in the end I concluded was just a bit too far out of my walking range. Five or six blocks at a time I might have been able to manage at my size, but not twelve or thirteen. So the walking habit was reluctantly surrendered once again in favour of driving to work instead. And sure enough, just like in 1998 when I first started driving to work, the weight slowly began to creep back up once more ...

* * *

Two years later, all that I had lost in 2010 had returned with interest. By January 2015 I had reached 137kg; in pounds, I had broken the 300 mark for the first time. At 175cm tall, this translated to a staggeringly high Body Mass Index (BMI) of 45.

My favourite shirt at this time was a size 6XL, and it was my favourite for that reason; 5XLs weren't really comfortable enough for me any more in the summer heat. My dress pants had a waist of 132cm, and they too were tight, the fabric between the thighs wearing thin as my legs constantly brushed against one another while walking.

During a visit to stay with my elder sister's family, her five-year-old daughter had told me straight up one evening: 'You're fat.' I smiled and told her she was right. Children in general terrify me, but one thing that I do admire about them is their tendency to say it like it is, before they reach an age where such honesty has been trained out of them in favour of understanding what is and isn't considered socially acceptable.

She was, of course, simply telling the truth as she saw it. To suggest that I looked like Fat Bastard from the *Austin Powers* movies would not have been an exaggeration. But as bad as I looked at this point, I probably felt even worse. The earlier loneliness and fear were long gone at this stage, but in their place now was workplace stress.

The end of 2014 was another trying time for me, as I had been struggling to balance too many priorities with too few people and too little time. I felt like the Christmas/New Year break was a complete waste, like I should have kept working through that holiday period. It was hard not to think about work all the time with so much still to do.

By the last weekend of that break I had literally worried myself sick. I could feel a familiar pain developing in my chest and, just like 2009, it felt worse when trying to lie down to sleep. So just like last time, I gave the toll-free Healthline number a call, they referred me to an ambulance and I was taken for another ride to the hospital.

I was sure to mention my previous hospital stay in Christchurch, and that this adventure physically felt a lot to me like that one. Given the earlier diagnosis of pericarditis, they focused their initial checks in that area with another ECG, a chest X-ray and so on. But once again, little turned up that they saw as being out of the ordinary, and for a while I feared they would discharge me that very evening. But the pain was real, and I begged them to let me stay overnight just so I could at least get one more good night's sleep, in a bed that could be raised on an angle. Thankfully they relented, taking some blood for more overnight tests.

The following morning, however, the results came back more or less all clear. Just like last time, apart from being fat and in pain, there apparently wasn't anything all that wrong with me. Well, I sure felt pretty wrong, but okay. These were the experts in their field, after all. So I was sent home armed with yet more ibuprofen and orders to stay away from work for another week.

During that week off I made an appointment to see a doctor in Dunedin for the first time, the latest addition to a long line of different doctors that I'd seen between all of the different places at which I'd lived over the years. Some of them had been quite friendly and personable, others somewhat less diplomatic in their assessment with comments such as: 'Are you aware of just how overweight you are?' Gosh, you don't say?

This one lay somewhere in the middle of that spectrum. After explaining my recent hospital stay to him, he had a look through my record and decided that I needed to be tested for a few more things, and gave me a slip of paper with instructions for the lab to take some blood for this, this, and this, plus this and that. 'I'd like to get you checked for diabetes,' he explained, 'then we'll see what we can do about … that,' motioning to my stomach like it was going to be no big deal to sort out. Yeah, right.

The diabetes prospect was scary, though. I didn't need any more health problems to worry about; being fat on its own had always been more than enough. That lab sheet stayed buried at the bottom of my bag until I eventually forgot about it. The next time I found it weeks later, it had been stained and crumpled beyond the point of usefulness. I felt guilty for not having done what I was told, but the fear of a fresh new diagnosis was just too great.

Back at work, I discussed my situation with some of my colleagues there. One made mention of a time when she was diagnosed with costochondritis; could that have been the source of my pain, as opposed to pericarditis? Whatever it was, it sure felt like something-itis, anyway. Something was definitely not feeling right in that chest area.

Another colleague suggested I try some physiotherapy. His partner ran a clinic in town, and helpfully organised a few appointments to see what they could do for me. I had a couple of chest massage sessions there while lying on my back and always felt better after one of those. Attempting some back massage was tricky though, as that meant lying on my stomach, which was something that by now I hadn't been able to do comfortably for many years, as it was just too big.

One day to my surprise, they wheeled in what appeared to be the perfect solution to my problem: another bed with a strategically placed hole through the middle of it. Here I could lie relatively flat on my front, letting my stomach just hang naturally through the hole as required. 'This is genius,' I told them. 'Do you do a lot of work with overweight types?'

'Well, we do a bit of work with pregnant women, and usually we break this out for them.'

Oh dear. While I have to admit I felt physically quite comfortable lying in that position on that bed, I was plumbing fresh new depths of shame in doing so.

For all the benefits that the various forms of physio did provide, the ibuprofen was a lot cheaper. But the relief that both treatments provided was only temporary. As soon as I would run out of ibuprofen, the chest pain would return. That was a worry. Is this the point where I would have to start taking medication for the rest of my life, still in my mid-30s? I was too young for that sort of thing just yet, surely.

And yet, deep down, a part of me figured that maybe this was going to be it for me, that this is how it all starts. It does say on the back of the packet, after all, that ibuprofen is not something that's supposed to be taken for the long term. So what would I do for the pain when ibuprofen would no longer be an allowable option for me?

On the other hand, though, if ibuprofen is only supposed to be a short-term solution, then perhaps it was never the right treatment for me in the first place? Could it be that it was not actually treating the cause of my pain, but merely the symptom of the pain itself? If that were true, then surely there would be other options for me anyway, to address the actual underlying cause of the pain?

So I went back to my doctor. Neither of us made mention of his previous prescription, but this time, he wanted to refer me to a dietitian.

Hahahaha, no. 'What the hell would the point of that be?' I barked. 'I'll just be told to eat less, and move more. Cut the calories, eat less fat. All hail the food pyramid. Seriously, I've been there, I've done all that. You can try to refer me if you like, but I can tell you now I won't be going. It didn't work then, it won't work now. Just give me whatever else you can instead, please.'

So it was back to the ibuprofen once again.

In the continuing search for a better solution, I re-examined my earlier decision not to walk to work. For a couple of days in 2014 it had snowed to the point where it was no longer safe to drive. I'd had no choice but to walk in on those days, and it was about as difficult as I'd expected it would be. I remember lumbering in on one of those snowy mornings, arriving a breathless, sweaty mess. A colleague was surprised to see me. 'Did you walk all the way in?'

'Yeah,' I huffed.

'Nice. So is this the start of some sort of new routine of yours?'

'Hah, no way.'

'Oh,' she replied with a hint of disappointment, before bravely asking her next question. 'Why not?'

'Because I'd rather die at fifty-five than at thirty-five,' I shot back.

This was a fair reflection of my attitude at that time. For most of my adult life I'd continued along the path of inevitability I had first mapped out for myself so long ago: I would die alone and before my time. Walking that distance to work at that size was just too hard, which was why I had chosen to drive again in the first place. I would if I could, but I can't so I shan't.

But then it occurred to me one day that perhaps part of the reason for the difficulty was the weather conditions. What if it hadn't been icy or snowing? What if it was dry? Perhaps it would be easier if I tried walking in on a normal day instead?

And so, in the short week following Easter of 2015, I finally took up the challenge of walking to work on a regular basis once again, a distance of about 2.5km (or 1.5 miles) in each direction. The timing here was very deliberate; in my mind, the only thing worse than a physical struggle was to be seen by others to be physically struggling. But with the days getting shorter and the nights getting longer, it would mean that most of the walking would be done under the cover of darkness, for the next few months at least, anyway.

I did it every day that it didn't rain, which usually amounted to three or four times a week. And as it turned out, it was indeed slightly easier in better weather, though still by no means easy in absolute terms. It usually took me a good 45 minutes in each direction, longer on the way home since I needed to climb half a hill coming back. By the time I staggered through the front door, I'd be so exhausted that I would turn on the TV and just flop down in the chair for another 45 minutes afterwards to recover.

For all that effort, the weight did at least begin, however gradually, to start to work its way backwards again. The chest pain, though, was still not improving. I felt as if my body was only barely capable of coping with itself in its current state. But still I pushed on, if nothing else so that if the worst were to happen, nobody could claim that I had sat back and simply allowed it to happen. 'Here lies Brendan,' I imagined the words on my tombstone. 'At least he tried.'

After a couple of months of this hard slog, I ran into further difficulty with my breathing, for which even the ibuprofen didn't seem to be enough any more, so yet another visit to the doctor beckoned. My regular doctor happened to be away that day, however, so I saw someone different instead. She suggested something I didn't expect, referring me to another nearby physiotherapist who specialised in breathing techniques. This was something new. A bit weird maybe, but new. Worth a shot.

I met this physio a few days later, and she began by asking me to tell her a bit about myself and why I was there. She seemed to be paying close attention to what I was saying, when in fact she was paying even more attention to how I was saying it. When I'd finished, she pointed out the extent to which I'd been using my chest to breathe, instead of my belly. Apparently I'd been breathing wrong my entire life, without realising it. How does that even happen?

The memory stirred, and then echoed, over and over. 'Suck in your gut ... suck in your gut ...' The one piece of advice I'd received as a child that I thought was actually helpful, and even that turned out to be a mistake that I would now have to let go. Sigh.

It took a few sessions over the course of a few weeks, but I slowly learned to relax my belly muscles and breathe differently. Naturally my clothes seemed to shrink another size again along the way, but that was all that clothes had ever done on me anyway, so what else was new?

Well, here was something new. One sunny Saturday morning a couple of weeks later, I woke up and the chest pain was gone, out of the blue, just like that. And that sure felt good. Great even, to be both pain-free and med-free for the first time in six months.

This feeling of freedom returned was an important leg up that got me thinking some more. By July I was down to 134.5kg. Since the walking thing seemed to be working, perhaps I could just exercise my way out of this? I mean, it was only working barely, but soft drink experiment aside, that was still better than any diet I had tried before. Everyone says it's all about diet and exercise, but my experience seemed to suggest otherwise, so maybe I just needed to go hard out on the exercise alone?

I mulled over that one for a long time, mindful of all the difficulty that I'd been through when I was younger. But maybe as an adult, I would at least have the power to say no to anything that I felt I just couldn't do. I felt like now was the time for me to seek professional help on this. So for the first time in my life, I decided I would do something that I once vowed I would never do: I would make an appointment at a gym.

I did the research from home and considered the options. Anything near work was written out of the equation immediately, as a couple of colleagues already did the gym thing at lunchtime, and it was absolutely vital that no-one would find out I was even thinking about this. Anywhere that sold themselves too hard was eliminated as well. If I'm going to do this, I don't want to stand out any more than was absolutely necessary.

Eventually I picked out a gym that appeared to have a more rehabilitative image about it. It also happened to be the closest one to home and the furthest from work. Surely I wouldn't run into any familiar faces there. If anybody I knew found out what I was doing, I would just bury myself in shame forever.

It took me an hour to write an email just a few lines long, and it took me the rest of the day to click Send. I deliberately sent it on a Sunday, so that I wouldn't be drawn into any silly little game of checking my email every few minutes for the whole day.

The reply came early the following morning, and an appointment was officially set for the following week. I booked some annual leave for the afternoon itself, only telling people that I had an appointment in town, and only if they asked. This was my secret, and mine only. No-one needs to know. No-one can *ever* know.

Finally the day arrived. It was a sunny but cool Monday afternoon in October. I'd walked past the place a couple of times previously, so I already knew where to go. In I went, and parked myself in the waiting area while warm sweaty bodies of various shapes and sizes — but always smaller than me, of course — occasionally drifted past in various directions. The problem with gyms, I mused, is that they're full of people who don't really need to be going to gyms.

After a few minutes the manager emerged, we shook hands and I followed him nervously towards the hallway. Then just as we rounded the corner before his office, I walked right into my aunt from across town, just as she was leaving.

Our reactions to each other were polar opposites. In the exact same moment that her face lit up in pleasant surprise, my heart plunged. I'd known that she was a gym-goer, but I'd had no idea specifically where she went. Of all the times that I could have found this out. This, needless to say, was a disaster.

It was all I could do to swear her to secrecy on the spot, before sitting down with the gym manager in his office. There in my now clearly distressed state, I rambled through much of what I've written in this book so far from the beginning. I threw myself upon the mercy of the court. I'd come this far, so I may as well see it through.

His response was the last thing I expected. 'There's nothing I can do for you here,' he said. 'Sure, I could sign you up to a membership and you might lose ten kilos or so, but you won't sustain it. You need a longer-term solution that you can maintain by yourself. Let's look at your diet. What are you eating?'

Oh, this wasn't going to end well. 'Whatever I want, and the answer to your next question is, because eating what I was told to eat while growing up didn't change a thing. Diets are all the same, none of them work.'

'I bet you haven't tried this.' He brought up a website on his computer, called the *Real Meal Revolution*.[2] 'Just watch these videos and take the quiz. Look, you can eat bacon and eggs and still lose weight.'

I hate bacon and eggs. 'This reads like Atkins,' I observed, thinking back to those news stories from the early 2000s. 'Wasn't that discredited years ago?'

'Mate, I've been in this business for more than twenty years, and I've seen plenty of people just like you come through my doors,' he explained. 'I wouldn't be where I am today if I didn't have some idea of how to help these people, and I'm telling you, this is the best thing for you right now. You said it yourself, you've been this way your entire life, what's the worst that could happen by just trying it?'

'Everything I've already been through before, all over again,' I retorted. 'I'm sorry, this isn't what I came looking for.'

His frustration began to show. 'All right, I'll tell you what. As you know, normally there's a fee for your first consultation here. I will waive that fee for you today right here, right now, if you promise me you'll try this. That's how sure I am about it. If it doesn't work, then forget about it. No harm done. And if it does work, you can come back and pay me later?'

Well, at least this wasn't going to cost me any money any more. After a short stare-off, I sighed and gave him my word. I didn't even really mean it at the time, I just wanted to get out.

I stormed the rest of the way home in a rage. After all that planning and effort to arrange this secret meeting to sort my life out, having convinced myself that exercise was the only solution, only to be discovered by someone I knew before it even began, and then to be told to go all the way back to square one and change my diet instead?

It was all too much. In the absolute depths of my despair, I cried that night for the first time in my adult life.

* * *

For the next few days my physical life was just going through the motions and nothing more. I got up, ate, went to work, worked a while, ate, worked some more, went home, ate, went to bed. But mentally, I was trapped in this continuous loop of reasoning, devoting every available ounce of brainpower that I had to work it all through.

Gym Guy is telling me to go completely against the official guidelines, to do something that everybody else says will kill me. But the guidelines can't be wrong because ... well, they're the guidelines. So Gym Guy must be wrong. But he said it himself, he's had 20 years of experience helping people like me for a living. He has to have a clue about something. But if he's right, then that means the guidelines must be wrong. But the guidelines can't be wrong because ...

... and so on.

By Thursday of that week I decided I'd had enough of that line of thinking, and took a step back for a moment. To this point in my life, I'd done everything that everyone had ever told me to do, and it hadn't worked. Why should this guy be any different? I still couldn't quite bring myself to believe him on this basis.

But then I weighed up the alternative, to *not* take his advice. And it occurred to me then for the first time. I do actually have a choice here. But is it a choice between two options that won't work, or a choice between one option that I know won't work, and another option that I *don't* know won't work? Can I really afford to assume that what he's saying won't work, just because nothing else has?

It was like that scene in *The Matrix*, when Neo is about to step out of the car into the rain, and Trinity warns him not to. 'You've been down that road before. You know exactly where it ends. And I know that's not where you want to be.' That was true enough.

The gears began to grind some more. If Gym Guy is telling me to go against the guidelines, then this has to therefore mean that one of them must be wrong. On the balance of probabilities, it just had to be him. But until I actually try following his advice, I cannot know for sure exactly how wrong he is. He was right about that much at least; surely it couldn't hurt to just try, if nothing else just to prove how wrong he really was.

And so that's when I dared to go and look up the Real Meal Revolution website for the first time. Wait, I have to pay for this online course? So this is going to cost me money after all? Hah. No, hang on, the first week is free. Hmmm. Well, I could just sit and watch the first couple of videos, I suppose. No-one needs to know.

The first video was less than two minutes long, and consisted of a simple introduction to Professor Tim Noakes from Cape Town, South Africa, a.k.a. the 'Prof'. As the saying goes, first impressions are everything, and I have to say I felt a pretty good vibe here. He seemed happy, warm and genuine in his work, presenting himself respectfully to his audience without being hard-sell at all. It was enough to get me to start watching the next video, at least.

That one changed everything.

This video was called *The Obesity Myth*. It began by explaining how various groups of humans across history and around the world all evolved on variations of a low-carbohydrate, high-fat (LCHF) diet, so it was therefore reasonable to expect that it wouldn't do any harm, because if it did, then we probably wouldn't still be here as a species. Fair enough, I supposed.

It then proposed that the current standard Western diet established over the course of the 20th century — but particularly since the 1970s with the development of dietary guidelines and the healthy food pyramid — is the real cause of today's diabetes and obesity epidemic, since our bodies simply aren't designed to process many of the kinds of foods that we are now being directed to eat.

Wait a minute. You mean to tell me that the healthy food pyramid — the basis upon which all previous dietary advice had been prescribed to me throughout my life — was wrong? That was a shock, but it was the right sort of shock to keep me watching.

I then learned about something called insulin resistance, a condition that manifests when the body is forced to constantly produce elevated levels of insulin in response to high blood sugar levels, which in turn are caused primarily by eating carbohydrates. I was effectively being told that if I ate too many carbs for my level of insulin resistance, then I would get fat; therefore, in order to lose weight, I had to cut the carbs. That was when I first began to really connect with the whole LCHF concept; it neatly explained why some people get fat eating certain foods, but others don't. And since it can also be inherited, that explained why I was particularly susceptible, because it also ran in my family to some degree.

Wow. I gave myself the rest of the evening to take in what I had just watched. I felt like I needed it. What am I being led into here? I'd heard of insulin before, but I thought that related to diabetes and not obesity, and certainly I'd never heard of this idea of insulin resistance. Having said that, my doctor had wanted to test me for diabetes. Could this really all be true? I wondered if I needed to cross-reference some of this stuff, but even without yet having done so, everything that the Prof was telling me seemed to be making fair and reasonable sense on its own merits thus far.

I felt a bit like how I would feel when somebody was trying to teach me some secret new strategy in a video game. It was taking a while to wrap my brain around it all, but on the strength of the extent to which I could currently understand it, I wanted to learn more. Perhaps I would never sufficiently understand it without actually giving it a go for myself, but we'd cross that bridge when we come to it.

The following evening I watched all of the remaining free videos. One explained the differences between good fats and bad fats, and the last was all about shopping and how to read food labels. Now there was some knowledge that I could immediately test for myself. I got up and looked at the food labels on everything I had in my cupboards, my fridge and my freezer. How many carbs per 100g was I eating? Various frozen pizzas, pies, noodles, even good old trusty bread suddenly didn't look so trusty any more: 20g, 30g, 40g. My jar of strawberry jam read 65g/100g, all of which was sugar.

Okay, so ... let's assume, just for argument's sake, that there might actually be some merit behind this low-carb idea. How could I possibly apply the idea in practice?

The website urged me to restrict my carb intake to no more than 5g of net carbs per 100g of food, but I was afraid I wouldn't find enough items at the supermarket that were that low, so I planned to allow myself up to 10g for starters. Using the 'green list' of recommended foods on the website as a guide, I wrote up my first ever shopping list, which I have kept to this day:

- 3L water bottle
- cranberry juice (unsweetened)
- burger patties
- lettuce
- eggs
- black pepper
- salmon
- canned tuna
- chicken breast
- steak
- mince
- milk (whole)
- cottage cheese
- vegetable soup

Not a perfect list of course, but there would be plenty more to come.

It was the longest shop that I had done in a while, since I hardly knew where to even find a lot of these things at first. I was zig-zagging all over the place, stopping each time to check the food labels. It almost felt like some kind of fetch quest from a video game: 'Go forth and collect any yonder items with sufficiently low carb content. Beware of dragons.'

It must have taken me half the day, but I had half the day to spare. I remember being disappointed at not being able to grab several old favourites any more, but there were other more pleasant surprises. Cheddar cheese: yes! Spam: yes, I haven't had that in years. Mushrooms: oh yeah, I do like them, I didn't think to add those. Stir-fry veges: hmmm, they would go well with the chicken breast if I cut that up ...

I got home with all of these new-fangled groceries with the realisation that I had now reached a point of no return. Now that I had all of this stuff, somehow I needed to figure out how I was going to eat all of this stuff. And not only that, but where would I find the time to learn how to prepare all of this stuff?

The game I was spending most of my spare time playing at this point was *Guild Wars 2*. I'd been playing it fairly solidly since its release in 2012, and now an expansion for the game was about to be released. This should have been exciting news, except that in this particular instance, many upcoming changes were proving unpopular with a number of players, myself included. Some aspects of the game that I greatly enjoyed were being removed entirely. For me, the game seemed like it was about to become a whole lot worse.

Was it going to be bad enough for me to stop playing on its own merits? Hard to say for certain. But when combined with the need for more time in the real world in order to take this low-carb thing seriously, it was a fairly straightforward decision to at least take a break from the game for a while. Suddenly, my evenings would be free again. I'd have all the time I would ever need to figure out this whole kitchen business. There was simply no reason left not to.

My very first low-carb meal was a couple of bunless burgers for lunch. The day was Saturday the 17th of October 2015. I weighed 132kg/291lb.

And so the stage was set for the showdown of a lifetime: it was me versus the Gym Guy. One way or another, somebody's dietary beliefs were bound to be exposed. One way or another, somebody here was going down.

5   THE JOURNEY, PART 1

At times the world may seem an unfriendly and sinister place, but believe
that there is much more good in it than bad. All you have to do is look hard
enough, and what might seem to be a series of unfortunate events may in
fact be the first steps of a journey.

—*Lemony Snicket,* A Series of Unfortunate Events, *1999–2006*[1]

'Hey, Brendan?'

'Yeah?' I answered, still staring straight ahead at my screen for a
moment, before turning my head towards the voice behind me to my
left.

I heard the click before I realised where it came from. My
colleague was holding his phone and had just taken a picture of me
at my desk, surrounded by a total of four fans arrayed in various
positions, all blowing at me full tilt. It was an unseasonably warm day
outside, and in an office with no meaningful air conditioning system,
that meant an uncomfortably warm day inside, especially for the
resident fatty.

I still hated my picture being taken, for still obvious reasons. But I
was able to see the humour in this particular situation, so I was still
able to laugh it off easily enough. At least, until the photo was then

emailed around the office with the subject line: 'Brendan is hot'. That part took a little longer to get over.

It was meant well, but what nobody knew at the time was that, less than a week earlier, I had just committed to trying low carb for the first time. It was late October 2015, I was still 132kg as far as I knew — having not yet dared to weigh myself since that first bunless burger — and so my confidence was still desperately vulnerable.

Even as I was getting under way, I had to admit that I still wasn't completely sure if I could do this. I still found it hard to shake the nagging feeling that, since nothing else had ever worked for me previously, this shouldn't turn out any differently either. From my position, it was an easy assumption to make.

One important realisation I made very early on was that whatever happens, if this was to somehow actually work, it would need to be something that I could sustain. Gym Guy was right about that, I decided. Even if taking things at my own pace meant that it would take me years to get to where I wanted to be, that would still be better than if I went too hard and burned myself out halfway there. I should always feel capable of taking the next step, to do it not just today but again tomorrow, wherever I might be up to along the way. It shouldn't feel too hard at any point.

Of course, I still needed to balance the need for sustainability with the desire for results. So I decided to set a few ground rules for myself, some boundaries that I wanted to learn to live within, to ensure that I would continue to take this sufficiently seriously — but not excessively seriously — along the way. For me to be able to genuinely prove Gym Guy wrong, I had to be giving this an honest shot.

The first rule was that I would never, ever go hungry. A large part of me believed that I was surely setting myself up for failure here. Going hungry seemed to be just one of those perfectly acceptable ideas that people trying to lose weight were always supposed to just have to get used to, yet for me, it had always led to my downfall. Well, screw that. If I'm to sustain this, I need to be satisfied following my meals. If I still have to continue to starve myself, then this ain't going to happen.

The second rule — as per the end of the previous chapter — was that I would limit my carbohydrate intake as much as I possibly could, since that was clearly the foundation of this dietary approach, but while still maintaining enough food variety so that I wouldn't die of boredom along the way. To start off with, I would only allow food that contained no more than 10g of carbohydrate per 100g according to the label. I don't care what it is, if it's low in carbs, I'm going to try it.

The third rule was that I wanted to achieve some tangible results; I had to see some actual weight loss. This perhaps sounds a bit silly on its own, but considering how ineffective past dieting attempts had been for me, I didn't think it was too much to ask. At the end of the day, this was the reason for doing anything at all. If the scales weren't going to co-operate, then neither would I.

My new routine evolved very gradually. I didn't feel I could go cold turkey and just toss out all of the bread and pizza that I still had in the house, so I continued to eat from the options I had available to me at first. Technically yes, this would constitute an immediate violation of Rule Two, but in my defence, I really felt like I needed the time to learn how best to prepare all of these new foods that I was supposed to be transitioning to, anyway. As long as I stuck to buying the good stuff, I would eventually say goodbye to each of the bad old things as I finished them off, and would hopefully replace them with further new food ideas going forward, as I would discover them.

Rule One on the other hand was easy to follow. I still had breakfast, lunch and dinner every day, and snacked in between as often as I felt the need. While the nature of what I was eating was beginning to change, the frequency of my eating was not; my appetite would simply not permit anything less.

Rule Three posed a bit of a dilemma, however, as I soon realised that I hadn't actually set a timeframe for my intended weight loss. I hadn't set any specific goals beyond 'this just has to work.' Goal setting was quite difficult for me at first, because I'd never known what it was like to be anything other than fat, so I honestly had no idea of what I was capable of becoming. So at first I didn't weigh myself at all. This was as much out of fear as anything else; I was so afraid that this wasn't going to work, that I was actually scared of proving myself right if I weighed myself too soon.

I finally conquered that fear about three weeks in, and couldn't believe my eyes as I discovered I'd lost 2kg in that time. I hadn't lost weight that quickly since giving up soft drinks in 2010. Could Gym Guy have actually been on to something here? Nah, it's too soon to know. Early days yet, let's see how things continue.

The website recommended that I keep a food diary. No way, I thought, that sounded like a lot of effort. But I soon developed a similar habit for myself instead: the shopping list. Not only would I write one up across the week before the next supermarket visit, but I would also keep each one afterwards as a reference. They were what I would be eating from anyway, at least once the last of the bad old stuff was gone. From here on, I would continue to maintain a small pile of shopping lists going forward, maybe a few months' worth at a time.

One of the first challenges at home was breakfast. Prof Noakes was all about the eggs in his videos, but I'd just never been a fan of the taste of them, and so consequently I'd never really even learned how to cook them. But I knew someone who had.

And so for the first time, I voluntarily let someone into what was until then a circle of one, when I contacted my brother to ask him for ideas on how best to cook eggs. Considering that he knew how much I hated eggs as much as I knew how much he loved them, his momentary brain explosion was pretty fun to watch. Once he regathered himself, he suggested that I just grate some cheese into them to add a little flavour, then scramble them in the microwave for a few minutes. I later added some sausage to the plate as well, to what would soon become my new breakfast staple.

The habits had begun to change at home, but I was still eating out a lot during the day while I was at work. I recognised that sooner or later, things would have to change there too. So one Friday lunchtime over a burger and fries at the local grill, I broke the news to two of my closest colleagues.

Like I'd done with my brother, I framed it to the guys as an idea, an experiment, but one that I wanted to take fairly seriously, and so it was for that reason that I wouldn't be able to frequent many of our regular lunch spots any more. No more pizza, no more curry, no more fried rice, no more burgers and fries ... after today, of course. As I recall, it was a pretty good burger that day too, but perhaps I was just really savouring it with the knowledge that it would also be my last.

This plan was something that I was prepared to commit to, with or without their support. I was honestly expecting to be going without it, as I assumed that they wouldn't want to give up their usual options purely for my sake, so it came as a pleasant surprise when they happily agreed to go along with it. From now on, whenever we would go to lunch together, it would have to be somewhere that included a suitable option for me. And of course when it was just the two of them, they could still go wherever they wanted.

By November the food transition process was almost complete. I'd run out of most of the bad old stuff at home, with just a few things left over at this point. There was an unopened jar of strawberry jam and two cans of spaghetti that I was able to donate to the annual workplace Christmas food donation drive. Beyond that was just most of a loaf of bread and half a tub of margarine, both of which in the end I finally threw out. That simple act was a minor accomplishment in its own right, as I recognised that my need to be eating right had finally overcome my need to not let anything go to waste.

In their place I was beginning to figure out a few new dinner options for myself. The first few were mostly bunless burgers, stir-fry vegetables with chicken or a simple can of vege soup. Things like mince or steak I would sometimes just have by itself, and even that was a challenge to get right for a kitchen newbie like me. I still had a lot to learn and I knew it, but for the time being, I still wanted to learn as well, certainly for as long as the scales would continue to show me favour, as per Rule Three.

And show me favour they continued to do. After seven weeks I'd lost 6kg.

I'd heard about how some people experience various symptoms while in their first few weeks of a low-carb diet, but for me so far it had been relatively painless. Maybe it helped that my transition had been a gradual one, I don't know. I did pick up on a metallic taste in my mouth at times accompanied by a little bad breath, which for a while was enough for me to worry that other people in the office might notice. But if they did, nobody had said so, and it was soon on the way out again anyway.

By now I was also encouraged enough to begin weighing myself daily. This was an attempt to observe any possible reaction following each day's set of meals, to make sure that I wasn't making any overly obvious mistakes. Which was just as well, as I certainly made a few here and there.

My usual lunch spot had become a nearby cafeteria that had a different buffet menu every day. Each week they would send out an email with the following week's full menu offerings; this was great as it allowed me to plan my dinners as well, to ensure that they in turn would be different from my lunches.

One day for lunch they offered pizza and vegetables. But when I turned up, it turned out that of all things, they had somehow run out of vegetables, but not pizza. I still wasn't going to go hungry though, so for the sake of Rule One, I decided to again violate Rule Two and filled up on what was there. When weighing myself at home afterwards, I immediately noticed that the scales now refused to budge. They didn't rebound, but they definitely stopped for a while before eventually resuming their downward crawl once again. That mistake cost me about three or four days of weight loss, effectively half a kilogram or about a pound. Lesson learned.

It was now December 2015, and I'd paid for and completed the full beginner's course through the Real Meal Revolution website. I'd been going at it for long enough now and had seen enough progress by now to have been fully convinced that this was going to be something worth sticking to, so I began to set some goals for the first time:

- Get to 120kg sometime in January 2016, which was my weight when I left high school.
- Get to 110kg by the end of April 2016, after around six months of low carb.
- Get to 100kg by October 2016, a full year after I'd started.

The latter two were entirely speculative; I truly had no idea where I was going to end up with this. I figured it was likely that I would level off naturally over time at some point, but to ever reach a weight approaching normal was still surely a bridge too far. Here lay the difference between my hopes and my dreams: I had never stopped dreaming, but I had given up all hope so long ago. It felt positively strange to begin to have that hope again, so I tried to be careful not to get too far ahead of myself.

My first big social test since switching to low carb came in the lead-up to Christmas when my aunt — the same one who caught me that day at the gym — invited my cousins and me to a family catch-up dinner. I'd lost 9kg in 10 weeks at this point. The potatoes were passed around the table, they reached me, I passed them along and ... no-one seemed to care. She did ask me about it afterwards, but thankfully chose her moment when no-one else was around. One of my cousins also told me she thought I'd looked better. That was important to me, that someone had noticed — seemingly unprompted — for the first time. That made things seem more real somehow.

For a long time I'd always been very grinchy around annual social occasions such as Christmas, but historically I did mark the day in my own way by making a great big trifle, which would take me two or three days to eat by myself. But this time around I was worried about the consequences of the sugar in all that lemonade and jam, so I skipped Christmas even more so than usual: this time I skipped it completely. No sweet treats whatsoever, just another regular week of eating instead. My reward that week was another kilogram gone and, sure enough, two weeks into January I reached 120kg. To be able to say that I hadn't been this 'small' since high school, that felt pretty good.

My clothes were slowly becoming more comfortable, then too comfortable, then too loose. By now I was finally beginning to drift backwards through my wardrobe, fitting into a few things that I hadn't worn in a while. I thought about all of the clothes I'd outgrown over the years, many of which I'd long since thrown out by this point, but I still had a few items to aim for. Wouldn't it be great if one day I was finally able to properly fit that bright yellow polo shirt at the far end?

In the meantime, though, my gradual downsizing still had to be accommodated along the way. During a New Year's sale in the first week of January, I went clothes shopping and found myself walking out with smaller clothes for the first time, ever. This could hopefully be the beginning of an exciting new trend, I thought. More and more, it was becoming apparent to me that that Saturday in October might well have been — to borrow from *Clerks II* — the first day of the rest of my life.

* * *

With the 2016 new year came renewed determination, and a desire for more knowledge. I watched through all of the various recipe videos on the website. Most of them were still too complicated for me; anything beyond just a handful of ingredients was still enough to put me off. But I was impressed by the simplicity of omelettes, as well as their versatility in terms of what I could fill them with. Grated cheese was always going to be a given, but I also tried various combinations of chopped spam or sausages, cherry tomatoes and mushrooms, before eventually settling on a preferred combination of cheese and half a can of tuna.

Having consumed just about the entirety of the website at this point, I then ordered the *Real Meal Revolution* book online,[2] and read the whole thing in a single weekend when it arrived. There were more recipes in the book too, including another sufficiently simple one involving fried salmon with spinach. That would make a nice addition to my dinner rotation, I thought. I'd already begun looking around online for information on which vegetables were considered the most nutrient-dense, and spinach was one that regularly appeared near the top of many lists.

I also started looking around online for more videos to watch, not just from Prof Noakes but from any other name that kept appearing regularly in my search results. Surely he can't be the only one out there promoting low carb; it would be great to finally be able to properly cross-reference his information with some other sources, and maybe branch out a little.

The very first online video that I watched following a reference from the Real Meal Revolution website was a TEDx Talk by Dr Sarah Hallberg called *Reversing Type 2 Diabetes Starts with Ignoring the Guidelines*.[3] Diabetes wasn't so much my issue — at least not as far as I was aware — but obesity was discussed just as much, and the two conditions were able to be tied together through that same underlying metabolic mechanism that Prof Noakes had first introduced me to: insulin resistance. This seemed like a good start.

Another name that I soon latched on to was Dr Stephen Phinney, whose various presentations on *The Art and Science of Low Carbohydrate Living* really convinced me not to be afraid of the right kinds of fat.[4] Prof Noakes had said the same thing in his videos, but the idea of fully embracing fat again after being told for so long that it would be literally the worst possible thing I could eat, was a mental hurdle that took some overcoming.

Not that all fat was universally okay, they said. Monounsaturated fats were supposed to be fine, as were saturated fats apparently, to my surprise. Some polyunsaturated fats needed to be kept under control, though, mainly those that came in the form of processed vegetable oils. That was interesting, I thought, glancing at my bottle of canola oil perched above the stove, complete with its red tick on the front of the label, the New

Zealand Heart Foundation's officially designated seal of approval at the time.

Still, neither Noakes nor Phinney had done me any wrong when it came to carbs, so I felt that I could trust them when it came to fat as well. Accordingly, when the canola oil ran out, I simply began frying in butter. When the last of my processed cheese slices ran out, I simply bought bigger blocks of cheddar. I phased out cottage cheese in favour of sour cream. I began to add aioli to my weekly plate of salmon and spinach. I sought out the fattiest cuts of steak at the supermarket that I could find.

This all seemed to help kick my weight loss into a new gear, and I somehow lost 6kg across the month of January to reach 116kg. What made that feat all the more impressive was that I had made another mistake along the way; when my usual lunchtime buffet option was closed one day, I fell back to one of my old haunts and had myself a plate of beef fried rice. And once again, just like they'd done with the pizza earlier, the scales halted for another half a week or so. But blip aside, the overall direction was looking good.

My previous doctor also moved on that month, and was replaced by another. I checked in with him and the first thing he asked me when I walked in was: 'How's the chest?' He'd clearly been prepping for me by going over the notes from his predecessor. I was pleased to tell him that that was all ancient history now, that I was starting to lose some meaningful amount of weight and that I was motivated to keep doing what I was doing. He said he was pleased to hear it, though I wondered if I still read a degree of scepticism in his voice. That would have been fair enough though, I thought. He hadn't seen me before then, and I was still huge by anyone's standards. Never mind, I'll show him too.

One day in early February, I discovered a half-rotten banana stuck to the bottom of my backpack that I carried to work each day. Gross! How on earth could I have let that happen? I used to snack between meals all the time. What's going on here? I could only guess that I just hadn't felt the need to snack between meals for so long, that it had just sat in my bag ever since I'd first put it there. I didn't think much of it at first, beyond the unpleasant job of having to clean it up, of course.

Later that month, I was having lunch with one of my colleagues at the cafeteria. I don't remember what was on the buffet menu that day, but I do remember the occasion particularly well for another reason. The day was bright and sunny. I had finished my plate and, like I'd always done before, I moved to get up for seconds. A buffet is all-you-can-eat, after all. But then I sat back down again as I realised that I didn't actually feel like eating any more. One plate alone was enough to fill me up. I couldn't believe it!

Then I began to connect the dots. My appetite had already begun to fall away, without my even realising it. It had started with the snacking, which would explain how that banana came to stay in my bag for so long that it went rotten. And now it seemed I'd reached the point where it was starting to affect my main meals as well.

I hadn't read about this phenomenon before now, but I was keen to find out if the low-carb diet had anything to do with it. And sure enough, a quick search online revealed that eating low carb can indeed lead to a natural reduction in appetite over time.[5] It made sense to me on reflection, that if my body was finally recognising that I was already carrying fat to burn, then there wouldn't be so much of a need to feed it externally any more.

This was a pivotal moment in my journey as I finally realised that this was how low carb could be reconciled with one key element of traditional dietary advice. For so long I'd always been told to just eat less, but with the focus having always been on fat, since fat is more energy dense then either protein or carbohydrate. That had never worked out for me in the long run though, because I'd always just gotten hungry.

Yet now, having cut the carbs instead of the fat, I found that it was becoming easier to eat less overall. I was needing less food to fill me up, and I was able to stay full for longer. But best of all was that it felt totally natural, completely effortless and thus, it seemed like this was going to be perfectly sustainable. This was happening by itself, without my having to go to any great trouble at all. That oftenfantasised scenario from my primary school days of being able to live off my own fat stores was finally actually beginning to happen. How exciting!

From here on out I would start to pay much more attention to how hungry I was feeling at mealtimes. I started to learn to really listen to my body and stop eating when I was full, rather than continue eating just because it was on the plate in front of me. I was still eating whenever I was hungry, still following Rule One, but now I was needing less in order to still follow that rule.

There were also further tweaks to the diet itself during February, though not so much in terms of food variety. I began to compare food labels, not just between different foods, but between different brands of the same foods. This came from an idea of mine that I could possibly reduce my carb intake even further — as per Rule Two — without impacting on total variety, by simply swapping brands of some existing foods from one to another.

To my pleasant surprise, there was indeed room for further improvement with this approach. My original burger patties were 9.6g carbs per 100g, for example, and then I swapped to others that were 4.1g. There were other smaller improvements as well with different brands of vege soup, sour cream and so on. By the end of the month, the only thing in my kitchen that still contained more than 5g/100g was a bottle of 'low sugar' tomato sauce, at 16g. With each item swap, I was getting closer to the Real Meal Revolution's original proposal of staying under 5g/100g across the board.

In addition to delving into the details with food labels, I was also watching the scales more closely, now weighing myself twice daily. This was frequently enough to spot another pattern, as I soon noticed that I tended to weigh less in the mornings than in the evenings. Rather than a constant gradual weight loss over time, it seemed as if it was all coming off overnight and then mostly coming back on again across the day, with only the net daily differences accumulating into longer-term weight loss. I supposed that made sense in a way, given that I was eating across the day and not when I was asleep, but I didn't expect the degree of intra-daily variation that I was seeing.

More people were starting to notice the difference in my outward appearance by now as well. Some were telling me about conversations they'd had with others about how well I'd been doing, all of which was wonderful to hear. After decades of being put down for my appearance, I was finally being complimented for it for the first time in my life. This was hugely uplifting for my confidence, providing all the motivation I would ever need to stay the course.

Even my father noticed when I visited him later in February for the first time since I'd begun low carbing, having lost a total of 19kg in 18 weeks at that point to have reached 113kg. His response was typically laconic: 'Oh, you've lost a chin.' Nice one, Dad.

One day in early March while randomly surfing the web at work during my lunch hour, I found a link to a low-carb support forum. Now there's an idea, I thought to myself. This could be a great outlet for me, without having to bother too many other people in real life with the various details of my journey.

That night I registered. As part of the registration process I had to think about my goals some more; here everything was expressed in pounds, not kilograms. Out came the converter. It looks like I started in October at about 291 pounds; now, what to enter for a final goal weight? I punched in a few various numbers, and settled on 191. That would be a loss of exactly 100 pounds, or roughly 45kg, and would take me to 87kg, a full 50kg from my peak weight. 87kg also roughly marked the point where I would officially drop from 'obese' to 'overweight' on the BMI scale. So that would do for now.

I soon posted a self-introduction on the forum as was the tradition there, not quite knowing what to expect in response. But right from the start, I was welcomed with open arms. In fact, the very first question asked of me was if I was familiar with fellow New Zealanders Prof Grant Schofield and Dr Caryn Zinn? I'd watched a couple of presentations by Dr Zinn at that point, and I knew that both she and Prof Schofield were based at the Auckland University of Technology (AUT), but that was about as far as it went. Still, the fact that they were also known to people overseas, encouraged me to start following them both a little more closely in the future.

For the moment, though, I was still working through my Phinney phase. I was impressed enough with his videos at this point to decide that I needed to purchase some of his writing. I found a number of positive reviews about two books that he had co-authored: *The Art and Science of Low Carbohydrate Living* with Dr Jeff Volek,[6] and *The New Atkins for a New You* with both Dr Volek and Dr Eric Westman.[7] Seeing the Atkins name again also piqued my interest; I remembered drawing the comparison of the Real Meal Revolution with my understanding of what the Atkins diet was, during my meeting with Gym Guy last year. In the end I ordered a copy of both.

The dietary evolution continued over the following weeks while I waited for those books to arrive. I tried experimenting with some kale in place of the spinach that usually went with my fried salmon, and one week when neither could be found at the supermarket, I picked up some bok choy instead. While I didn't mind either substitute — particularly their extra crispiness when coming out of the pan — I decided I preferred the taste of spinach overall.

I'd heard much by this time about the benefits of avocado. Many fruits were off limits to me by virtue of their carb count being over 10g/100g, but avocados were both low in carbs and high in fat: literally LCHF. But I was disappointed in their taste when I tried them. Maybe they could serve as a kind of snack food with a little salt added? But then, I hardly needed to snack any more anyway. So they were given a miss.

I'd also read about how a lot of people like to make substitutes for certain foods that were no longer allowed under LCHF, for example, mashed potato. I suppose I could admit to missing potatoes a little bit, but that was vastly outweighed by the fact that I now knew they were just too starchy for me, so I never missed them to the extent that I had any great urge to try making a direct substitute. If anything, I might have worried that having a substitute might make me miss the original even more.

Nevertheless, curiosity took hold when I read that cauliflower could be mashed as a substitute for potato. This could potentially be something to go with my occasional steak and mushrooms, I decided.

So one day I bought my first cauliflower, fully intent on mashing it for dinner until I discovered that I didn't actually have a potato masher either. So the next day on the way home from work, I bought my first potato masher as well. And in the end, this change would indeed turn out to be one that would stick.

Finally during the month of March, I hit my original April goal of 110kg, a full six weeks ahead of my original schedule, and bringing my total weight loss through LCHF to 51 pounds. That put me just over the halfway mark to the goal that I had only recently set on the forum a couple of weeks earlier.

I didn't really feel in my mind like my journey was halfway over already, but the numbers were certainly welcomed, all the same. One thing was becoming clear to me by now though: Gym Guy had been right all along, after all.

* * *

Around the middle of March 2016 I decided to start a journal. I hadn't really bothered to start one any sooner as I'd never really felt like I'd needed to. But now, I'd reached the stage where I actually wanted to. I'd come far enough to this point to want to be sure that my efforts wouldn't someday go to waste, and so a journal to me felt like a good way to keep both my thoughts and my actions well on track as the journey continued. 'I still have a long way to go, of course,' I wrote on the 19th, 'but certainly things have fallen into place well enough for me so far, to really believe that I can get there one day.'

That same late summer's day I had attended that year's local comic book convention, where I had the pleasure of meeting and being photographed alongside former WWE pro-wrestler Haku, as well as Marina Sirtis who played Counsellor Deanna Troi in *Star Trek: The Next Generation*. The latter photo came out particularly well by my standards; I mean, I still didn't exactly like what I saw, but I hated it less than usual. At least my neck wasn't quite as wide as my head any more.

By this time I weighed around 109kg. Considering that I'd now lost 23kg since the previous October, I might have expected to see more of a physical difference than I did. Thinking about this some more, I eventually took the view that it all came down to percentages; while a person going from 130kg to 120kg loses the same amount as someone going from 90kg to 80kg, in percentage terms the first is nothing like the second. So even just by maintaining this general trend of losing roughly 1kg per week, the rate of change from a visual perspective would actually accelerate, the longer I'd go. That was a very exciting thought!

To say that my kitchen skills were improving by the beginning of April would have been a bit of an overstatement, as this would imply that I had kitchen skills of any great degree to begin with. Perhaps a better way to put it would be that I was starting to 'fail less'.

My cauli-mash began to approach something resembling edibility. After the water was drained I would mash in some butter, then some grated cheese, a shake of salt and plenty of pepper, the latter of which reminded me of my Nana, who always loved pepper in her mashed potatoes when I was young.

Following the purchase of a masher the previous month, April also saw the introduction of another implement that I'd never even heard of, until I'd encountered a few recipes that required the use of one: a spiraliser, something like a giant pencil sharpener but for vegetables, which could turn them into noodles. I tried it with cucumber at first, with the aim of adding the noodles to the mince, but they came out pretty watery. Later on I would switch to courgettes instead, which worked better.

The support forum continued to offer plenty of other new food ideas as well, and for a while I was able to maintain a trend of coming home from the supermarket each week armed with one new thing for me to try. This was me taking full advantage of Rule Two for variety's sake: if it's low in carbs, I wanted to try it.

One week I bought a jar of olives. My only experience with olives to this point had been as a pizza topping, and they weren't amongst my favourite choices, so this was a bit of a gamble. And sure enough, this particular gamble did not pay off. Never mind.

A key point that I picked up from *New Atkins* was the concept of a 'carb ladder', with each rung representing foods with an increased level of carbs. To date I'd been enjoying plenty of the first two rungs, with a little bit of rung number four in the form of fruit, mainly berries. But the third rung was all about nuts, which I hadn't considered at all until then. So after checking various labels in the aisle, I picked up a small bag each of hazelnuts and macadamia nuts. The former went down okay, but the latter … oh my. Discoveries like this were what made the whole exploration process worthwhile! The night that first bag of macadamias was finished, I made a special trip back to the supermarket just to buy two more.

Another week I picked up some asparagus, following a suggestion that I could wrap the shoots in slices of prosciutto and then bake them in the oven. They came out all right, but I found them to be a bit bland for an entire meal. Maybe just a few at a time for a snack, but then I wasn't snacking so much any more anyway, so that one didn't quite manage to stick.

And then there was coconut. My expectations going into that particular experiment were fairly low, since I'd never quite enjoyed coconut-flavoured … anything really, so why should I expect to take a liking to the real thing? As it turned out, I rather enjoyed the taste of fresh coconut water, and didn't mind the flesh too much either. But my problem turned out to be the sheer amount of effort involved in trying to crack them open: way off the chart, well into my 'can't be bothered' territory in this instance. Well, at least now I knew.

Finally, I introduced myself to konjac/shirataki noodles after finally finding a packet at the supermarket. I had them with mince and tomatoes, almost like a fake spaghetti bolognese. Unfortunately, however, I didn't really care for their jelly-like texture, and I was worried if I kept having them, that — just like the earlier cauli-mash experiment going in — I would start to miss the real thing more.

Food wasn't the only thing being tried and devoured, as I continued to consume whatever low-carb literature I could find along the way too. Once I'd finished *New Atkins*, I picked up a copy of *What the Fat?* by Grant Schofield, Caryn Zinn and Craig Rodger.[8] And I think what I appreciated most about this book was its simple, plain English, practical approach to incorporating LCHF into one's daily life. This only served to validate my earlier curiosity in these fellow Kiwis.

Then finally it was back to Drs Volek and Phinney for *The Art and Science of Low Carbohydrate Living*. And boy, was that one a winner. I wasn't able to fully grasp all of the details during the first read, but that was part of what made it so interesting. What I did understand though made perfect sense, and what I didn't ... well, that would be reason enough to read through it a second time one day.

One weekend in early April I took a trip to catch up with my sister whom I hadn't seen for a while. We had a good long chat, talking about the contents of my fridge and the various vegetables and other things that it now contained. She observed that many were things that neither of us had been fed as children: we never ate spinach, bok choy, broccoli or mushrooms while growing up, and even tomatoes were rare. But we had plenty of peas, beans, carrots, corn and, of course, potatoes; all of which were considerably more starchy than the veges I was eating now.

She hadn't known in advance what I'd been doing, so it was a pleasant surprise for her to have seen me the way I was at that point, now just over 107kg. And she wasn't the only one in for a shock either; when I caught up with another aunt of mine from Australia, she too was, in her own words, 'blown away.' Another evening I bumped into a former colleague while walking home, and even he noticed, despite my wearing a thicker jacket that night as the weather was beginning to cool.

That daily walk to work and back was slowly becoming easier, too. But then, I suppose anything becomes easier when one is no longer lugging around an extra 30kg like I was a year or so earlier, when the walking first began. And I have to admit, I enjoyed the little buzz of actually passing someone on the footpath every once in a while, even if most of them might have been ambling along with their faces buried in their phones. But hey, it was still better than what I'd been capable of doing before.

When I reported my improving physical ability to my forum friends, they congratulated me on my 'NSV', which I didn't understand at first, but soon came to learn that it stood for 'Non-Scale Victory'. This was something more typically attributed to achievements like fitting smaller clothes, but it still applied well enough here.

But it wasn't like there was any shortage of achievements in the clothing department to celebrate by this time, either. The drift backwards through my old wardrobe was well advanced by now. For so long I'd felt a bit weird for hanging on to as much older clothing as I'd done for so many years, but despite my wardrobe clear-out from a few years earlier, I still had enough left over to feel grateful that I hadn't thrown out even more. That investment was finally beginning to pay off now; it meant not having to spend quite so much on the way down.

There were a couple of drops of jeans sizes, each punctuated with several new belt notch reductions along the way. Whenever I debuted a smaller shirt at work, one or two colleagues would typically comment on how well it fitted me. It doesn't get much more real than that.

One day I rediscovered my old pair of dress pants that I thought I'd thrown out, since I'd actually worn holes into the inner thighs. They were what I'd been wearing a year ago, just before I started walking regularly. I checked their size, and the difference between them and the jeans I was wearing at this point was a full 30cm. That meant I'd lost an entire foot around my waist in about a year.

In coming to terms with the fact that I was actually on track to reversing this lifelong process of continual weight gain, I felt a bit like I'd stumbled into some sort of bizarro-world alternate universe, where rain falls up and the sun rises in the west, and that there was another me out there who was just going to keep going the way I always had been.

Looking at myself in the mirror, I remember thinking that the person staring back at me didn't really look like me any more. And I knew it was going to take some time to get used to, since I was still shrinking at a good rate. As I'd told a work colleague a couple of months prior: 'I don't know what I look like, under all this, I mean. Nobody does, and nobody really can.' I still didn't know even now, but I was well on my way to finding out, and I was looking forward to meeting that new me.

But there were still emotions in need of processing. I didn't feel particularly brave about how I'd more or less been keeping things to myself, only letting people in on what I was doing, as I felt comfortable. I still felt a certain sense of vulnerability about things even now; I had become fiercely protective of my new routine, even turning down some social opportunities, lest I found myself trapped in a situation that I wouldn't be prepared to deal with.

How some people from my past would react when they found out what I was doing, was not something that I was looking forward to, either. I grew up in the same small town for 20 years and I could easily imagine what a lot of those people would say, the next time I'd go back: 'See, I was right all along; all you needed to do was diet and exercise, what took you so long?' But I'll cross that bridge when I come to it, I decided.

The 17th of April 2016 marked exactly six months to the day since I had first started low carbing. On that day I took stock in my journal: 'I've lost fractionally over 26kg, from 132kg to just under 106kg, but I'm happy to just round it off so I can say I've lost an average of exactly 1kg/week over 26 weeks.'

What I found interesting at this point was comparing these last six months with the six months prior. During the previous six months across the winter of 2015, I'd lost 5kg just by walking to work and back. But in the six months between then and now, I'd lost more than five times that amount with a low-carb diet added to the walking. The difference between walking alone and walking plus low carb came to 21kg.

That appeared to make low carb approximately four times more effective than the walking by itself. Or to put it another way, around 81% of my weight loss was coming from low carb, versus 19% for exercise. People describe the concept of an 80/20 rule in various situations; it seemed to be applying pretty well here for me.

I hadn't written anything at all about my low-carb journey in social media thus far. In part, this was because I worried that I could lose control of the situation if too many people found out what was going on. Knowledge creates expectation, and expectation creates pressure. There was also a sense of fear that people might ridicule the means more than they would celebrate the ends. But as I was now at my halfway point in terms of my earlier time-based goals, I felt that a halfway-type announcement might be useful, as a test for the bigger reveal to come.

So to mark the occasion, I made the decision to 'go public' with my journey to date with a couple of my other old gaming communities, just to see how people there might respond.

The following morning I was delighted to read the replies, all of which were unanimous in their support:

'That's ... awesome, man. I love when people are legitimately happy and excited about changes they've made to their life. This might just inspire me to start really working out again.'

'Amazing to hear, thanks for sharing! I have to say it's very uplifting to hear how well you've been doing since you've given yourself all this time away from the game. I hope that everything continues to sail smoothly so you can reach your reward with a great deal of happiness and confidence to go with it.'

'Keep on keeping on. Staying in shape takes a lot of willpower and it seems like you got the jump you needed. Without a doubt, that is an amazing weight loss transformation. I can't say I've known anyone in real life who has had that much of an amazing turnover. Don't give up!'

'Well done! That's freaking awesome! Coincidentally my husband and I started LCHF end of January. He's lost 35lbs and I've lost 20lbs. I'm a big fan of LCHF as it's been the only thing that has ever worked for me. Have you been on dietdoctor.com at all? That's our favourite website next to the Fathead Facebook group.'

'That is so totally amazing! Good for you! I know first-hand how well that diet works. My husband was having issues with his breathing at night (terrible sleep apnoea) and issues with his heart as well. It scared him into getting really serious about his weight, and so we changed what we ate. He dropped about 60-ish pounds over the next six months, and got down to his high school graduation weight. Of course I lost weight too. Oh, and all his health problems? Gone. Even his doctor was shocked at the change. It really does work.'

Not a single smart-arse troll to be found, which — considering the audience in this case was a bunch of anonymous internet gamers — I thought was all the more remarkable. None of them questioned the approach. All they cared about were the results. All they cared about was that it worked.

The last two replies in particular got me thinking some more. 'There seems to be this simmering undercurrent of awareness out there among some of the general public that low carb really is a thing, regardless of what official guidelines might otherwise recommend,' I wrote in my journal later that morning. 'Maybe one day between us all, we'll reach this critical mass of "laypeople" whom the "experts" will simply no longer be able to deny ...'

6 THE JOURNEY, PART 2

You never know what's around the corner. It could be everything. Or it
could be nothing. You keep putting one foot in front of the other, and then
one day you look back and you've climbed a mountain.
 —*Tom Hiddleston*[1]

'SO, HOW LONG UNTIL YOU DISAPPEAR?'

Fortunately the question came before dinner was actually served,
otherwise I might have choked on something in my laughter.

I was across town, catching up with my aunt and uncle that
evening. There weren't so many others around this time, so it was
easier to discuss the subject a little more freely, keeping in mind the
fact that I still hadn't gone fully public with what I was doing.

For the record, the answer to the question would have been in
about two years at the going rate of roughly 1kg/2.2lb per week,
though I imagined I would be pretty happy with wherever I might
end up after another five or six months.

April had now become May, and by the 5th of that month I had
reached 102kg. This marked another milestone as I had now lost
exactly 30kg since I'd started low carbing less than seven months
earlier. 'It's kind of a lot,' I wrote in my journal the following

weekend. 'I'm now at the sort of weight that I used to dream about, as if it could never possibly happen. Still a fatty though of course, but just a bit less so now.'

Even then with all that I'd lost to that point, I still found it hard to imagine me not being fat, as that was simply all I'd ever known for my entire life. To date, my 'normal' had been for me to be very 'different' from the rest. So to me, the idea of actually being of a normal weight was, ironically, very different.

As I approached my original October goal of 100kg, thoughts began to turn towards a re-evaluation of those earlier goals. Where might I expect to end up now? When I first joined the support forum back in March, I'd settled on the idea of losing 100lb in total, but with no specific timeframe in mind. Maybe if I joined those two ideas together? 100 pounds translated back into 45kg, so that would take me to 87kg by October. Sounds like a plan, I decided.

My forum friends had been nothing sort of wonderful in cheering me on with each new milestone. The fact that they tracked their weight in pounds was something I was able to turn into a positive of its own, despite personally being used to kilograms. Tracking my weight by both measures at once effectively meant double the number of milestones to celebrate along the way.

One common milestone that these people liked to celebrate was what they called 'onederland' (pronounced 'wonderland'), that being to dip below the 200-pound mark and into the 100s. I was still some way off from there at about 225lb myself, but I did put a related idea to the group: 'If going under 200 pounds is considered to be onederland,' I asked them, 'can going under 100kg be considered reaching nonederland?' And that sounded as good to them as it did to me.

The autumn of 2016 was a fairly short one, with temperatures remaining mostly mild well into May, at which point the weather suddenly turned and then stayed that way. By then I had entered into my third new belt and my fifth new pair of jeans. The daily walk to work and back was definitely becoming easier now as the new jeans were fitting me better all around, as opposed to what jeans used to be like for me: tight around the waist, loose around the legs. I could now take much bigger strides and not get caught up in myself, as it were.

Such Non-Scale Victories (NSVs) would leave behind them a trail of now-oversized clothing. With each new round of clothes shopping, I found myself needing to pack up the largest items from my existing range, for no other reason than I was simply running out of wardrobe space. No longer was I donating old clothes away because they were too small for me, now I was donating them because they were too big.

By the middle of May I'd already donated away four bags full, with plenty of other still-nice shirts beginning to accumulate at the bigger end of my wardrobe. I was getting closer to fitting everything at the smaller end now, although that bright yellow polo shirt from my radio days continued to lurk just out of reach for the time being. Never mind, all in good time.

As winter approached I tried some of last year's warmer clothes and was pleasantly surprised at how loosely everything was hanging. That prompted yet another day at the shops, just to see what was out there. In the end I came home with two polar fleeces and two pairs of trackpants. Their size: XL. And they were available in sizes from S up to 5XL. So now I was wearing clothes that were closer to their smallest available size than they were to their biggest. By this measure, it seemed that I was quite ... normal?

I was reminded of a conversation that I'd recently had with another work colleague. He'd simply told me straight out one day: 'You know, you don't really look all that fat any more. You did six months ago, but now you just look like a guy with a bit of a tummy, no worse than any of the rest of us.'

I hadn't necessarily agreed with him at the time, but it's amazing what each new round of smaller clothes does to one's self-confidence. 'I can't wait until the next time I get to go somewhere and be noticed now,' I wrote in my journal that evening. 'And to think I'm still nowhere near goal. Very exciting!'

Not every change was necessarily a happy one, though. At the end of May came clothing donation number five, but this time it meant saying goodbye to some real old friends, when I dropped off two old pairs of trackpants and a polar fleece top to the clothing bin. These were clothes that I'd worn every winter for the last 20 years, more than half of my life, but they were just way too big for me now and taking up space that was now needed by the newer stuff that I'd recently bought.

Of course I'd already thrown out plenty of other clothes by this point, but they were mostly work shirts and a few pairs of jeans. This time, however, it was comfortable casual home wear, the first time I'd let go of things that actually felt quite hard to do. How strange it was to feel so sentimental about clothes that I'd been ashamed of wearing all those years. 'So many memories of times spent wearing certain things,' I journaled that evening. 'Somehow I feel a bit older tonight.'

The longer nights of winter were perfect for doing a bit more reading. Top of my list at this time was *Why We Get Fat* by Gary Taubes,[2] which I found really compelling, although by this stage I had figured out most of the reasons for why I personally had gotten fat already. Maybe if I'd read this earlier, it wouldn't have taken me so long to come around to the idea of embracing LCHF in the first place.

Next up were a pair of low-carb cookbooks. Even now, I was still on the lookout for further food ideas that would help grow my overall meal variety. As per Rule Two, if it's low in carbs, I wanted to try it. Unfortunately I found myself to be outright intimidated by a number of the recipes, many of which came with long lists of exotic and/or expensive ingredients. Far too complicated for a kitchen noob like me; anything with a list of ingredients longer than about five would cause my brain to short circuit. Simplicity was still too important a factor in ensuring overall sustainability, as far as I was concerned.

Luckily, there were still some sufficiently simple discoveries out there, just waiting to be found. During another family catch-up weekend, we ate at the local Burger Fuel restaurant for lunch. I was a bit nervous about it at first, but I was assured that there were low-carb options there, and sure enough, I was able to request a low-carb version of any of their established burger options, where they replaced the buns with more lettuce. 'It's a shame there isn't a Burger Fuel in my town, as I'd be only too happy to add them to my rotation otherwise,' I wrote in my journal when I returned home.

I was also noticing a regular trend with another of my meal options. It seemed that whenever I would enjoy a dinner of salmon, spinach and aioli, I would typically find myself as much as a pound lighter the next morning. This phenomenon, I was told online, was called a 'whoosh', where weight is suddenly lost following a period of relative stability.

I was able to verify the status of this particular meal as a personal whoosh trigger of mine, by changing the nights of the week at which I would eat it. And it generally continued to pay dividends the following morning. When I tried having it more than once a week though to see if I could speed things along, that didn't appear to stack up. It was definitely proving a good option for me, but it was only good for once a week.

Speaking of weight loss, 'nonederland' was finally reached at the end of May, as my scales dipped below 100kg for the first time since my mid-teens, triggering another fresh round of online celebrations with my forum friends.

The following weekend in June I made a trip to see my father. The last time I travelled there was around the end of February when I weighed 113kg, but I was still wearing familiar clothes even if they had certainly loosened by then. But this time at 98.5kg/217lb, and with my new winter wardrobe that actually properly fitted me, Dad was pretty astounded at the difference. He even made the comment that he thought I looked taller.

I received a similar reaction just a few days prior as well, from a colleague who had recently returned to work after a year's maternity leave. I'm not sure my appearance had ever been described as 'amazing' by anyone before, so that was a nice first.

And yet, that word would be repeated in even more emphatic fashion the following week when, one morning on my way in to work I ran into my cousin, the same one from that dinner last Christmas who was the first to have noticed a change. She looked me up and down on the street corner there, and her revised assessment in front of all the other pedestrians was, and I quote: 'you look amazing, holy shit!'

As awkward as these moments sometimes were when receiving feedback like this, the words themselves were like gold dust to my brain that, for so long, had been bankrupt of positive thoughts where my body image was concerned. And I was continuing to pick up other small changes for myself along the way as well. 'It's nice to be able to spot something resembling a jawline now for pretty much the first time ever,' I wrote in my journal on the 9th of that month.

The walking continued to progress well. While the distance being covered each day was still the same, the time taken to cover it was continuing to improve. Conditions were good for a bit of a power walk on the way home one evening, so I left work at 5pm on the dot, and when I arrived home, the microwave clock read 5:31pm. That was pretty good, considering it used to take me closer to 45 minutes when I'd first started walking more than a year earlier. The traffic lights were favourable but not perfect, so I wondered if I could maybe make it home one day in under half an hour?

My forum friends, as always, were full of support and encouragement. Not only did they have complete faith that I could someday crack the half-hour mark, but they also had other exercise ideas for me.

One suggested that I try jogging, but I wasn't so sure about that. I couldn't help but feel very protective of my knees, mindful of the lifetime's worth of added pressure that they'd already been under for such a long time. It was even something of a running gag (no pun intended) with some of my work colleagues, who loved to call me out whenever I might dash quickly across the road.

Another suggested that I try planking and to look up some online videos for how it was done. I could see the appeal here; there were levels so easy that even I might be able to manage them, and it would only take a few minutes a day, with no investment required in any equipment. Something to experiment with in my own time, perhaps.

By the middle of June I had reached 97kg/214lb, which made it 35kg lost in as many weeks, and 40kg altogether when including the previous six months' worth of walking. It had now been eight months since I started low carbing, which meant I was now exactly two thirds of the way through this year-long chapter in my life.

It was at about this time that I considered yet another revision of my goals. It hadn't been very long since I'd already decided on a goal of 87kg/191lb by October, equating to a loss of 45kg/100lb within a year. But after losing an average of a kilo a week for so long, I wondered if maybe I was even capable of reaching 82kg/180lb at some point? That would mean losing a full 50kg on LCHF.

A half-century of kilos. That felt like such a massive number to be claiming to have lost. Still impossible to visualise, and yet I was only 15kg away at this point. Could it actually happen? There was only one way to find out.

Onwards and downwards ...

* * *

It was towards the end of June that I began to notice some people's reactions starting to evolve a little as I continued to shrink. Where everybody used to get excited at my progress, now in some cases they were starting to get a bit nervous as I began to approach their own weight.

It felt a bit like being an underdog in some sport or another, who picks up a series of unexpected wins, and along the way they gain support on the basis of their newfound winning streak. But those new supporters still have their old favourites, and it becomes a lot harder to maintain that type of support once the underdog is no longer an underdog, but now a genuine threat to their own.

It soon became something of a motivator for me at this point in my journey. In the early days it was just about proving Gym Guy wrong. From here on out it was becoming more about proving these other people wrong instead. Maybe it was all in my head, but I assumed that they were out there somewhere.

Not that I knew anyone who outright wanted to see me fail, but I was sure there were those who were silently predicting that I would.

And that was fair enough, to some extent. We all hear that the hardest part about losing weight is keeping it off afterwards, but then I still hadn't finished losing that weight yet, anyway. One step at a time.

Things were finally beginning to slow down by July, though. The number of weeks on LCHF had begun to creep ahead of the number of kilos lost for the first time. And I'd just reset my goals only a few weeks earlier as well! Typical. Well, it had to start happening sometime, I supposed. Two questions remained though: how long would it take before I levelled off completely? And where would my weight be by that point?

At least there were still a few more NSVs to be celebrated in the meantime. By now I had begun to phase in another smaller size of shirts, which meant more larger shirts to bag off to the donation bin. My 38" jeans were feeling loose enough for me to start thinking about looking for some 36s. And since I was in the depths of winter, I dug out a couple of old turtlenecks which had been too small for me for about a decade or so, and sure enough, they were suddenly too big for me now as well. So they'd also need replacing.

During the second weekend of July I went to have a look around a local science exhibition that had opened for a week, starting on the Saturday. I just had to test the people at the nutrition stand, where they had a bunch of different foods and I was supposed to guess how much sugar was in each of them. I warned them upfront that I was on a low-carb diet, before running through each item and declaring them 'safe, too much, too much, too much, too much, marginal.'

The marginal item — at 4.9g/100g — was a small carton of milk. 'Oh no, milk is fine,' they said. 'It's only got a little sugar in it, and it has other things in it too which are very good for anyone on a balanced diet.' Except, of course, I'd just told them that I was low carbing! Never mind. I wasn't up for an argument about it, so I just smiled and politely backed away.

As another part of the week-long event, there was also supposed to be a place where one could get a free blood glucose test. I hadn't had that measured for many years, but now there was a degree of curiosity about where things might sit after nearly nine months of low carb.

So I turned up on the day, and it turned out that the person qualified to do those tests was away sick for the entire week, so I couldn't get it done then after all. But they did suggest I get some proper blood work done at some point, just so that I'd know. Especially in light of the weight I had lost, by which they were pretty impressed when I told them about it.

In the end, all they were able to do was confirm my height (175cm/5' 9") and measure my weight (95kg/210lb), blood pressure (135/85) and heart rate, which was 88 at first, but then I had just come up a few flights of stairs. It was back into the 60s again soon enough.

While mulling over the idea of getting some further blood testing done, I finally became the proud owner of two new turtlenecks that fit me nicely after a couple of weeks of searching: one dark grey and one navy blue. Thick enough to wear on their own, not too thin that they looked like thermals, and not too thick to then not be able to wrap up in a jacket for my walking. Just right!

The 36" jeans that I'd ordered online had arrived as well, so I picked them up during the same lunch hour as with the turtlenecks, and then even went as far as to order some 34s as well, since they were on sale at 20% off.

Of course, going clothes shopping for lunch meant that I didn't have lunch itself at all that day. This felt like a bit of a problem by around 3pm, but by 6:30pm that evening, I wasn't feeling like dinner any more strongly than usual. While I'd previously thought about skipping a meal here and there, I hadn't considered going without lunch during the week, as I felt that my working days were probably a bit too long for me to be able to tolerate that without going hungry. And there was never going to be any conscious violating of Rule One, no matter what.

Still, it was reassuring to know that having to go without a meal every now and then wasn't going to be the end of the world. Being totally fat adapted meant my body now recognised that it could simply feast on itself for a while instead. A year ago I wouldn't have believed that was possible. How things had changed.

This realisation that my body really seemed to be at peace with itself was enough to finally spur me into making an appointment with my doctor, at which I finally requested — and to which he was glad to issue in response — an order for a standard blood panel.

This was all stuff that my previous doctor had wanted me to get done 18 months earlier, but I'd chickened out at the time for fear of what might have come back. I was still a bit nervous about it at this point, but it was easy to remind myself that whatever comes back now will no doubt look a lot better than what would have come back then, when I was still carrying so much more.

The blood was taken early the following morning, and I was told to expect the results in a couple of days. So it was a bit of a surprise when an email arrived later that same evening: the results were in already. Uh-oh, this can't be good, I thought. I opened the attachment fearing the worst, and this was what I found (translations via an online converter):[3]

- HbA1c: 31 mmol/mol (5.0%)
- Total cholesterol: 6.5 mmol/l (251 mg/dL)
- Triglyceride: 0.7 mmol/l (62 mg/dL)
- HDL cholesterol: 1.86 mmol/l (72 mg/dL)
- LDL cholesterol: 4.3 mmol/l (166 mg/dL)

So, not so bad after all, it would seem. My A1c, triglycerides and HDL all looked fine. My LDL was marked as being 'high', but with everything else in pretty good order, it seemed like a bit of an outlier. I'd only begun reading about how to decipher blood work, and had heard that LDL can often climb in people eating LCHF, but both my doctor and I took the practical point of view that it wasn't worth worrying about too much on its own right now, with everything else looking as good as it otherwise did,[4] although further tests might be useful for the future.

Further testing from the past might have been useful now as well,

I realised. I didn't completely regret having skipped that test from a year and a half ago, though, as I knew enough to know that in some circles — health or life insurance, for example — a diagnosis of something like diabetes could be hard to shake, even if all symptoms were later reversed. Still, it raised an interesting philosophical question: what's the difference between someone who may or may not have been diabetic 18 months ago but isn't now, and someone who was formally diagnosed as diabetic 18 months ago but isn't now?

Still working through what felt like a bit of a phase of getting everything tested, I also took a trip into town the following weekend for a hair follicle analysis. After a short while the results came back, and for the most part they agreed with my blood work, with a few exceptions; I came up a little light on a couple of vitamins and minerals, for example. I had to laugh, though, at the lady's reaction when my omega-3 came back looking good: 'Oh, that's weird, usually everyone's really lacking in that.' Hooray for salmon!

However, the big catch with this kind of work — which I was told only after I agreed to the cost, of course — is that the results were only really a snapshot of one's readings at that moment in time. Compared to blood markers like A1c, for example, the values were therefore not as meaningful. My readings could be completely different again the next day just by eating differently. So regardless of the accuracy of the findings, the findings themselves weren't necessarily very useful in the long term. Never mind.

By the end of July I was really pushing the power walking on the way home, as weather permitted. One evening I left work at 5:04pm and the microwave read 5:33pm on arrival; for the first time ever, I had finally made the trip in under half an hour.

One thing I noticed about the walk home on another evening earlier that week was that I was never passed along the way at all, not even once. Always the passer, never the passee. I couldn't remember that ever happening before. There was even a middle-aged lady walking two greyhounds up the final hill on the footpath opposite, and I beat her to the top even though she had a head start at the bottom. It felt really good to think back to how hard this all was even just a year ago, when the whole world was faster than me. What a turnaround!

The month was capped off wonderfully when on the 30th, the scales finally read 92kg/203lb. So I had now lost exactly 40kg since I started low carbing 41 weeks earlier, and a total of 45kg from my original peak of 137kg as of April last year. No doubt the half-century mark would be harder to reach as I had so much less left to lose at this point, but it was still worth chasing in my mind.

There was plenty written in my journal that day. 'It's amazing when I look at the difference between where I am now and photos from last year. I showed one to a couple of colleagues yesterday and they were equally surprised; even they don't remember me being that big any more. That's good in a way I guess, as it means they're getting used to this new almost-normal me, just as I'm starting to now as well.

'Even now, I look down as I type and I can see the blood vessels on the back of my hands, the shadows accentuated by the low angle of the winter sun as it fights to break through the cloud cover. It wasn't so long ago that my hands were just big fleshy mittens; not any more. It's great that my thighs don't chafe any more; my pants are much quieter now when I'm walking. It's great to have a jawline; I can wrap my outstretched hands around my neck and the fingers are touching. Everything right now just feels great.'

And the signs for the future were still good too. One night earlier that week, I had a craving for bunless burgers for the first time. I'd been making and eating them for more than nine months by now and had always enjoyed them, but I was all set to make something else when I decided that what I actually felt like that night was bunless burgers, so I made some of those instead.

To have lived this lifestyle to the point where I was actually getting cravings for it now, was incredibly exciting. Why would I ever go back?

* * *

Having been born in the region, I've been a Highlanders rugby fan for as long as there have been Highlanders. Some years had been better than others, but none was so great as in 2015 when they finally clinched their maiden Super Rugby title. 'I DON'T KNOW WHAT TO SAY,' I blurted on social media that night, 'BUT I KNOW I WANT TO SAY IT WITH CAPS LOCK.' (And yes, I was sober; I don't drink.)

They may have fallen short in their 2016 campaign, but they'd still done enough that year for me to want to pick up a shirt of theirs for myself one day. The only problem was that since I'd been shrinking for so long by this point, I really wasn't sure which size I would end up fitting in the long term.

I finally took a punt at the start of August when, after trying on a couple of sizes instore at the local mall, I decided I would buy one that was currently one size too small for me. This shirt would hopefully help me to visualise what my final weight — and shape — might actually be. If and when I chose to post an 'after' photo, whenever that may be, I wanted to be wearing this shirt.

It may not have seemed like much at the time, but after wondering for so long, I did consider it a minor milestone that I was finally starting to reach a point where I could imagine where I might possibly end up. Only now was I really starting to believe that the end could actually be within my sight, if still not quite yet within my grasp.

And, of course, it helped that whenever I needed reminding of that, all I now needed to do was ... just look down.

I tried the shirt on a few times across the week, and noticed that, in places such as around my shoulders and arms, it actually fit me fine already. But it was just too tight around the middle. Now granted, this was sportswear made for sportspeople, and I was definitely not one of those. But it did occur to me that, even if I continued shrinking at my current proportions, in time it might end up being comfortable in the middle, but then too big up top.

Perhaps it was finally time to start exploring other exercise options more seriously. I was already getting plenty of walking in each day, so something different to really focus on the core and upper body. Perhaps I ought to start planking? Perhaps ... perhaps it was finally time for a follow-up meeting with the Gym Guy?

That was a terrifying thought, to say the least. My first visit there the previous year had been one of the most daunting experiences of my entire life, even counting the earthquakes. But with the benefit of hindsight, it was now blindingly obvious as to who had been proven wrong about LCHF. And even if I didn't mean it when I gave him my word at the time, I felt a sense of obligation to keep it now. I owed him one.

And so, just like last time, I put together an email requesting a second appointment. It took me about three minutes to write, and about three days to send. And once again, the response came through and a date was set, this time towards the end of the month.

There were yet more milestones to celebrate between now and then, and every single pound counted for something. When I slipped below 92kg to 202 pounds, that marked my 100th pound lost since my original peak weight of 302lb. When I drew closer to 91kg/201lb, that now meant I had lost a full third of my body weight. At an even 200lb I was right on the edge of onederland, and also now just below 91kg, giving me a BMI of 29.7; for the first time that I could remember, I was no longer clinically obese.

It had also taken me almost the entire winter, but I finally finished *Good Calories, Bad Calories* by Gary Taubes.[5] This was written before *Why We Get Fat*, but the former was just so much bigger and more detailed that I had decided to read his books in this order instead. No regrets.

That month I also bought a copy of the documentary *The Big Fat Fix* by Donal O'Neill and Dr Aseem Malhotra,[6] during which much emphasis was made of the benefits of extra virgin olive oil and just real food in general. What I also got out of it personally was some ideas on exercise: they demonstrated some basic movements like holding a rock in your arms while squatting/balancing on a large fallen tree trunk. As someone whose upper body strength was even more lacking than my kitchen skills, this was good practical stuff for me.

As the day drew nearer, I decided that whatever was going to come out of this, it would not involve my getting a gym subscription. There were a couple of reasons for this, the first of which was about timing. I would have to go at either the beginning of the day or the end of the day, either on my way to or from work. And I didn't see myself sustaining that. But things like planking, push-ups or squats in the evenings at home when I'm by myself and no-one's looking, that felt more likely to me.

Which led to my second reason. I don't care what anyone says about people 'not staring' at unfit types in gyms, I would still feel extremely 'stareable' regardless. Sure, I'd listen to what he suggests — he obviously gave some pretty good advice last time around — but I still had to feel comfortable with whatever options that might be presented to me. Comfortable enough for me to want to do it not just today, but again tomorrow. And gyms just weren't that kind of environment for me, I felt.

As nervous as I was about the upcoming appointment, however, I still felt better whenever I caught a glimpse of myself in the glass of a shop window while walking through town. The bigger picture still looked pretty good overall. 'To no longer hate and fear the way I look as I always had done in the past, but to actually develop a sense of accomplishment and — dare I say it, pride — in one's own appearance; these are the sorts of feelings that I'm learning to enjoy for the first time,' I wrote in my journal. 'It's pretty neat.'

The last little confidence booster before the big day came the night before, when the scales drifted close enough to 90kg for me to claim 199lb. To the delight of my forum friends, I had reached the fabled onederland at last.

The timing of the appointment itself was first thing in the morning. Having to get up an hour early was mitigated easily enough by a correspondingly early retirement the night before, but my brain refused to let go of the morning's prospects, and so the sleep that I did get was fleeting at best.

As a teenager, I once refused the offer of a free immunisation booster injection because, even though I had accepted it would be good for me, I felt overwhelmed by the simple prospect of the pain of the jab (though I did eventually go through with it). Throughout the night I waged another similar such battle of knowledge versus instinct. The rational part of me understood full well that the key to the next steps of my journey would be found by returning to 'that place', but countering that was years of built-up instinct screaming at me: 'No! Gyms are bad! Must avoid! Do not want!'

It was a relief when the 5am alarm finally sounded, and the usual routine began. The forecast of all-day drizzle proved accurate, so I would need my wet weather jacket. The same one I wore to Round One 10 months ago, only now it was about five sizes too big for me. Well, at least it would make for an easier comparison on his part, I supposed.

In the damp Dunedin darkness I trundled down the hill from home before hanging a left, left again and lastly up the stairwell to the reception area. Ah yes, nothing like a flood of bad memories for one's self-confidence at such a vital time. Even at 7am there was music pumping, instructors instructing and poor sods gasping. And there I was, feeling as out of place as an iceberg in the Sahara. Patience, I had to keep telling myself, as I stared into the wall behind the empty reception desk, it will all be over soon.

Then came a familiar voice from behind. 'Brendan!' I turned and there he was. 'Oh my God, you look great! I can see it just in your face, you look so much better!'

I smiled and nodded weakly, shaking his hand. 'It's been a while.'

Into his office we went, with no surprises waiting for me around the corner this time. He sat down at his desk, and I removed my jacket to reveal the smallest shirt I'd had left at the far end of my wardrobe: one bright yellow polo shirt that I hadn't worn now for 20 years. Achievement: unlocked.

'So tell me,' he asked, 'how have you been?'

Once again, I told him everything. 'I want to apologise for any past negativity on my part,' I began. I told him how upset I was when I left that previous day, that his advice seemed to fly in the face of everything else I'd been told my entire life, and how could all of that have been wrong? And yet, I realised that the only way I could prove him wrong was to try it. I completed the online Real Meal Revolution course, I bought the book and read it in a single weekend. I began watching other videos online, I bought and read half a dozen more books. I joined a support forum. I started a journal. And all along the way, I'd managed to lose 41kg in 10 months.

'That's ... amazing,' he repeated more than once. 'I'm so proud of you, mate. And you should be, too. You've done an incredible thing: you've changed your life. Really, you have. You must feel great?' His eyes were wide with wonder.

'I feel ... better,' I conceded wryly.

'So what's next then, do you think?' He wanted me to say it for myself.

'Well, I figure some form of exercise, I suppose. But it has to be right for me. It has to be something I can manage to some degree from the outset, yet improve on with time. I don't think I want to come here regularly if I can help it, I'd rather some sort of routine I can manage in the privacy of my own home. What do you think?'

'I know just the thing.' He turned to his trusty computer and brought up a series of interval-based training videos that he had personally recorded and uploaded online over the course of the past few months.[7] 'I instruct the viewer as if they were right here with me, and there's a great big timer in the corner there so you can just watch it on your PC and go when the clock does.'

It all looked suitably simple to me. At least one video appeared to include some form of planking, which immediately reminded me of the planking discussion that I'd been reading on the support forum a few months earlier. I had to laugh as I realised then that this could really work, and that this time, I had come to that conclusion a whole lot more quickly than last time. 'You might not have much more to lose at this point anyway,' he suggested. 'I'd say about eighty-five kilos would be a good weight for you.'

'This looks good,' I decided, as he emailed me the links. 'I'll have to give it a shot. Thank you so much for everything.'

'No problem, mate, glad I could help. See you in another ten months, eh?' he grinned. Another handshake, then it was off to reception for the bill, and back out the door and down the stairs. I was still relieved to be out of there again, but where once there had been anger at what had just happened, now there was only optimism for the future.

I'll have to admit, I still haven't been able to form as regular an exercise habit to the extent that I might have liked since then, beyond the regular walking to work and back. To this day, any form of higher intensity exercise, strength or resistance training, remains my weakness, a work-on still outstanding. But I had at least learned what would best suit me to be doing, should that habit come to properly form someday.

And I did keep the promise to pay him back.

* * *

The arrival of September 2016 heralded the gradual onset of spring. The days had been getting longer for a while, but only now were they actually starting to get warmer. With my revised weight loss goals now creeping onto the radar, I began to think more about clothes shopping for the summer ahead.

Historically I'd never been that high on the whole concept, for obvious reasons. I was traditionally one of those guys who would sneak down to the far end of the big boys aisle in whatever department store I was in, grab the biggest thing I could find, and buy it just in the hope that I might fit it, regardless of what it might have looked like. I wouldn't even try it on in the store first; I was always paranoid about someone seeing me through some changing room camera somewhere: 'Hey everybody, get a load of this fat guy trying to fit something new!'

But now, here I was in the position of having some options for the first time around what to wear. I was just about ready to retire the last of my 2XL shirts by this point and drop down to XLs, depending on the brand.

Depending on the brand? I had choices?! This was absolutely

mind-blowing to me, that other people who have always had these sorts of choices available to them, seemed to take them for granted.

For the first time, I had the freedom to think about things like styles and colours. What did I like? What didn't I like? I simply wasn't used to ideas of such flagrant indulgence. I still grapple with it sometimes even now.

One trend that soon began to develop was a liking for T-shirts with geeky retro/gaming designs on them, that I felt reflected who I was and where I came from. Some people might express themselves with jewellery, others with tattoos, but for me my outlet was definitely turning out to be T-shirts, so it was quite an exciting time to explore the options on that basis.

Of course, another round of clothes shopping meant another wardrobe clear-out, and since it was now spring I was a little more ruthless with the current collection. This resulted in not one but three more bags full of clothes that were donated away one Sunday.

It occurred to me towards the end of the month that there wouldn't actually be much left of my original wardrobe by the time I was all done and dusted. I'd still have my beanie, gloves, scarf, maybe some old pairs of socks, oh and my old dressing gown that I hadn't been able to fit for more than 20 years, yet had somehow managed to hang around all this time. But pretty much everything else would have been completely replaced. 'I've probably bought more clothes in the last nine months than I have in the last nine years,' I noted in my journal one morning.

Come October, and the goal that I had originally set for myself on the support forum just over six months ago was finally reached: 87kg/191lb. I'd now lost 45kg/100lb in 50 weeks of LCHF, at an average of exactly 2lb per week during that time. And when adding the 5kg/11lb that I'd lost in the six months beforehand, that made a total of 50kg/111lb lost over 18 months.

That was cause enough for celebration, and a very public one at that. After wondering about what to say for so long before now, the moment was finally at hand for my big reveal on social media:

'Well it seems that word is starting to leak out, so I guess it's time to make this official.

'So here we are. After dropping 50kg over the last 18 months (45 of that in the last 12), I am no longer an obesity statistic for the first time in living memory. Yep.

'To all the so-called experts out there who for years continued to advise the likes of "eat less, move more", "calories in, calories out", "you are what you eat" or ever invoked the "healthy food pyramid": you have no idea how wrong you all were.

'To the rare few of you on the other hand who were right, and to everyone else for their support along the way: thank you.'

The post included my first 'after' mugshot, and some people commented that they hardly recognised me. To be honest, I felt the same to some extent myself. My cheeks had practically imploded into my jaw, to the point where I had begun shopping for new sunglasses, such was the extent to which my current pair didn't properly fit my face any more.

My goatee also seemed somewhat surplus to requirements. I thought back to my radio days when I first grew that horrible neckbeard, and the promise I'd made to myself that I would never go clean-shaven again until I was truly happy with the way I looked. Was I there yet? I couldn't say. I had only just met this new me for the first time. I needed more time to think about it and get used to things. So for now, it would stay.

Two weeks later in the middle of October, I marked my first full year of LCHF. During that time I'd dropped a total of 46kg/102lb, to have reached 86kg/189lb. In contrast to a fortnight earlier, my journal entry that day was one of quiet satisfaction. 'I've smashed goal after goal across the year, and while I didn't reach my final 82kg goal in that time, I'm still pretty happy to have come this far, to say the least.'

Maybe I would end up settling at around 85kg, as Gym Guy predicted. I still wanted to try and push on to 82kg anyway, though. The allure of a low-carb half-century was strong. How close could I get?

I'd had another occasion to skip lunch one day recently when I was invited by a client to join them, only to find that all they had on offer there were bread rolls, pastries and chocolate cake. 'Oh, I'm sorry,' she said, 'are you gluten-free?'

'Worse,' I grinned, 'low carb.'

'Oh okay, I've heard about that. How's it been working out for you?'

'Coming up to a year now and I've lost about forty-five kilos.'

I couldn't help but chuckle at her reaction as she took a moment to collect her jaw from the floor. And yet at the same time, I also recalled that this wasn't the first time where I'd skipped a meal now, seemingly without any great consequence.

The idea of fasting wasn't new to me. I'd already read about the work of Dr Jason Fung in this area more than once, both on the support forum and on *Diet Doctor*, another low-carb website to which I had recently subscribed.[8] To my uncertain brain, however, the concept had long sounded too similar to the old adage of eating less. It took me a while longer to come to grips with fasting as being not so much about eating less, as it was about eating less *often*.

Besides, I had already learned how to sustainably eat less to a good degree already, but it had always been within the boundaries defined by Rule One: never go hungry. To go for longer periods without eating would require that I put that rule to the test.

By November, though, I realised that I wasn't too far away from a daily 16:8 intermittent fasting routine anyway. My regular breakfast of scrambled eggs and sausages had slowly become more and more difficult to finish each morning, to the point where all I had at the bottom of the bowl now was a puddle of a single egg and just a few bites of sausage. Some mornings I even felt brave enough to swap the eggs out altogether for a couple of slices of cheese along with a few cherry tomatoes or macadamia nuts, to save on preparation time.

That month I reached 84kg/185lb. Some people were starting to tell me that I needed to stop now, that I was getting too skinny. I could see their point some days; as the weather continued to warm, my daily walks were now able to be done without the need for a jacket, but just a shirt on its own. And indeed, whenever I caught a glimpse of myself in the shop windows now and then, I clearly looked thinner now than I could ever remember being.

Others were asking me when I was going to start 'eating normally' again, and they tended to react with surprise when I would tell them 'probably never.' I figured that at some stage I might allow myself some crumbed meat and maybe some more fruit now and then, things like that. It would all depend on how my body responded to whatever else I might try.

But however it might respond, wherever my limits might be in terms of carb intake, I understood that I would need to stay within those limits — once I'd found them — from then on. I remembered the lessons I'd learned from a year or so earlier. Every time I'd indulged in a little pizza or fried rice, the progress would halt immediately. It was only cheating if I didn't get caught, but my body knew it every time. For me, there were no such things as cheats, there were only mistakes.

And besides, I still had one last goal to reach.

The final push was on through the month of December. I decided to stretch my daily fasting window a little, to take a few nibbles of cheese and nuts with me to have at work instead of before the walk in. Work itself — like most places at this time of year — was always plenty busy, but that was no bad thing this time around. Some days I was busy enough to forget to have my morning snack at all, and I would only realise at lunchtime that I'd missed it completely.

Still, the payoff was good. By the 11th of the month I was hovering at around 83kg. If I hoped to make it by the end of the year, I was going to be cutting it close.

My plans for this upcoming Christmas were identical to those of the previous year: nothing special whatsoever. The old trifle habit had long been banished to the history books by now. No more great big bowls of refrigerated sugar for me any more, ever.

My only real gripe from around this time, according to my journal, was that I seemed to be settling somewhere awkwardly between clothing sizes. 'Most of the XL shirts I wear are feeling a little loose, but the Ls I've already bought so far are still a little tight.

For now I'm sticking with the XL stuff as the looser fit will undoubtedly be more comfortable during these summer months.' From there, I hoped that I could maybe work my way into the Ls over next winter, and then hopefully stay at that size or thereabouts going forward.

There was one last bag of clothes for the clothing bin that month, as another fresh batch of T-shirts arrived at work shortly before the break-up for Christmas.

There was no journal entry for Christmas Day itself, always a day of strict hibernation for me, but I did note on Boxing Day that the scales were hovering ever closer to that half-century mark. Without work to stretch out the length of my days at that point, I was effectively able to maintain a solid 16:8 intermittent fast every day. I hoped that another five days of that would be enough to get this thing wrapped up by year's end.

And, indeed, it was on the morning of New Year's Eve itself, the very last day of 2016, when the scales touched 82kg/180lb at long last, for the first time in almost a quarter of a century.

'So 2016 has been quite the year,' I wrote modestly that afternoon, 'with 40kg lost during that time, to add to the 15kg I lost in 2015. The total lost — between the low carb diet and the walking — comes to 55kg or 122lb, over 21 months.'

The weight loss journey was now complete. And what a ride it had been. I'd come so far. As Gym Guy himself had said, I'd literally changed my life. And only now was the true scale of the change beginning to dawn upon me, in more ways than one.

Not only had I undergone this amazing physical transformation, but I also felt like I'd somehow reached this resting, default emotional state of contentment. It was a subtle change, but it was there. The lows of old didn't feel as low now as they used to. Every time something might go wrong, I could just look back at what had gone so very, very right over the course of the last year and a bit. I used to be a fat ginger nerd; now I was just a regular-sized, plain old ginger nerd. Fat, no more.

No doubt there were things in life that I would never have

considered possible before now, and yet, only now that I had finally achieved all of my weight loss goals, did I realise that I wasn't actually sure what those life experiences could even be. I'd been fat for so long that I'd never given any serious thought as to what I could accomplish for myself if I was thin, because I'd never seriously believed it could ever happen.

And yet, now it had. The seemingly impossible had finally come true. I felt so empowered. I could do anything.

Now it seemed, the world itself was my proverbial oyster ...

7 THE REWARDS

The very basic core of a man's living spirit is his passion for adventure.
The joy of life comes from our encounters with new experiences, and hence
there is no greater joy than to have an endlessly changing horizon, for each
day to have a new and different sun.
   —Jon Krakauer, Into the Wild, 1997[1]

IN 2010 MY brother relocated to the United States, and it was a sad time to see him go. We kept in touch online in the years since he left, but the hope was always that someday we'd meet each other once again. At first we weren't sure who would travel to whom, but eventually it was decided that I would be the one to do the travelling.

The idea first began to take shape during 2015. The plan would be that I'd head over at some point during 2016, during either April or October, when the seasonal differences between hemispheres wouldn't be too great. Of course, at that time I was still struggling with my health, so the thinking was that perhaps it needed to happen sooner rather than later, as I feared that before long, there might come a time when it would no longer be physically possible for me to travel at all.

But by the end of 2015 once the low carbing had begun to take hold and things were beginning to measurably turn around, we decided to put it off to October 2016 rather than April. That would give me an additional six months to see how much I could improve myself beforehand.

Over the course of those six months the plan for the trip evolved further as my youngest sister opted to join me, and the itinerary soon expanded with the addition of some stopover time in Los Angeles, Philadelphia and New York. For someone whose own international experience to date had amounted to a couple of trips to Australia (which isn't that far when you're from New Zealand), this trip was turning into a pretty big deal.

I booked three weeks of leave from work, easily the most I'd ever taken at one time. A few were concerned at my being away for so long, but others were insistent that I forget about work and not check my emails at all while on holiday. We agreed to a compromise: I wrapped up as much work as I could beforehand, and left as much information as possible on what I couldn't. That way I wouldn't feel so much of a need to check in, as I wouldn't have much to offer at that point, anyway.

On the day before I left I took a photo of my feet on the scales, pointing at 86kg. One of my big fears going into all of this was how I would cope with not having so much control of the food that would be put in front of me. I decided I would try to take a practical approach: I would look for low-carb stuff wherever it could be found, but not stress too much over what else I would have to eat around that. Whatever I might gain as a consequence, I wanted to believe that I could shake it off again soon enough once I'd returned.

The first thing I noticed after boarding each plane was how much extra belt strap I had to spare. I'd never quite needed an extender in the past, but I had always used the absolute fullest length of the strap available, and it was always tight. Now I had a good 30cm or more to spare, and I could use some of that for comfort. Imagine if I was still the way I was a year ago, I thought. This trip was going to be so much better now.

By sheer coincidence, it had turned out that the departure date of our trip had fallen precisely one year to the day since I'd started low carbing. One year to the day since those first homemade bunless burgers, my sister and I were crossing the Pacific Ocean having departed Auckland in the evening for an overnight flight.

Upon arrival in LA around lunchtime local time, I half-expected to be stopped at customs, on account of the fact that I looked so different to the photo in my passport. I'd only had it taken nine months earlier, but in that time I'd lost over 30kg. But we were waved through without any issue, and were soon on the road to the hotel.

Man, this place is big, I remember thinking in the car. The sun was bright, the sky was clear, and while we could see hills in places, the city otherwise appeared to stretch all the way to the horizon in just about every direction, and the roads were so wide that they felt perfectly capable of taking us all the way there and beyond, if we'd wished. It all looked and felt a bit to me like a very large Melbourne, which in turn had felt a bit to me like a very large Christchurch at that time. Way to make a guy feel small.

The hotel in LA served a complimentary buffet breakfast, but it was all bread, croissants, cereals, yoghurt, fruit and fruit juice, so I had little choice but to wear some of that. Dining around Hollywood was mixed up a bit, but most of the time meant trying all of the fast food chains that didn't feature in New Zealand, like In-N-Out Burger, for example. So I worked within those options, getting burgers on their own instead of full combos, chicken wings instead of tacos and so on. Hooters was where I discovered the joy of fried mozzarella sticks; probably not the perfect starter option, but likely still better for me than most.

On the morning of our planned visit to Disneyland, the day dawned grey and drizzly. This meant nothing to us, but to the locals it was quite a big deal. There were reports of minor traffic accidents all over the news, and the hashtag *#LArain* was said to be trending on Twitter. This was apparently the first precipitation of any amount in the area for several months.

Disneyland itself was fun, for the most part. The drizzle was no great impediment and, if anything, possibly helped keep the crowds down a little on the day. We tried various rides across the morning, and then had a good lunch of meat and veges at one of the on-site restaurants. Important tip for future visits: Space Mountain is not the easiest choice for a ride immediately after having eaten!

We covered a lot of the other touristy stuff in LA as well. Wandering the Walk of Fame along Hollywood Boulevard, the wax museum, a quick ride on the subway to Union Station and back. A tour of the Griffith Observatory, a short hike to the top of the ridge just in front of the Hollywood sign, a lazy afternoon through the local zoo.

The days were busy, but the evenings were no less enjoyable for the chance they gave us to relax afterwards. One evening the hotel had organised a local musician to perform song requests from the inner courtyard area beside the pool. I requested Pink Floyd's *Wish You Were Here*, for no reason other than it was the best song I could think of for an acoustic guitar. We sat from our balcony and just enjoyed the free and easy sounds as the large, still-warm sun sank low in front of us.

And, of course, who wouldn't turn down the opportunity for a pool dip in a place like LA? I had felt far too self-conscious to have gone swimming anywhere for far too long, but once it was dark, I did indeed dare to break out the brand new togs and had a quiet paddle in the night.

On to Philadelphia next, via Houston as the flights were significantly cheaper that way than direct from LA. My lingering memory of the airport at Houston was of watching the motorised carts ferrying both passengers and baggage along the hallways across the terminal. Some of those passengers were larger than I had ever been. I couldn't help but feel pity for them, in a way that only people who had ever been that way themselves could really understand.

Our arrival in Philadelphia was late, but the following morning's buffet breakfast at the hotel more than made up for it. In addition to much of what had also been served at LA, here they also served scrambled egg and these tiny little sausages which had a flavour to them that I'd never tasted before. They turned out to be turkey sausages, and they were delicious.

From there we took a train to New York. I hadn't ridden a train for many years, and I really enjoyed the change in pace from air travel, getting a closer look at some of the rural American countryside for the first time. Then as we approached NYC itself, we entered a tunnel and stayed underground for some time, all the way to our stop. Whatever our first sight of the city was going to be, it was surely going to be a full and immediate immersion.

Soon enough we disembarked to the station floor, collected our luggage and followed the exit signs up a wide set of stairs, with no idea of what to expect at the top. And then all of a sudden, we emerged to find ourselves right in the heart of midtown Manhattan on Seventh Avenue, outside the famous Madison Square Garden itself. Our New York experience had begun.

It took some time to get used to the level of constant sensory bombardment that only a metropolis as massive as this could ever make. The lights, the sounds, the people, the traffic. Everything seemed everywhere. Yet the relief upon checking into the hotel was fleeting; we only had three nights booked there and the first of them was only a few hours away. We wandered over to nearby Central Park to while away our first late afternoon, and mapped out our plans for the next two days that night.

Most of our first full day was covered by a bus tour that looped its way around mid- and downtown Manhattan. We had the freedom to hop on and off at various designated stops and could just catch the next bus on the loop when we were ready to move on.

Our first stop was outside the Empire State Building, where we joined the steady stream of tourists that appeared to be filing through the place. The floor number inside the elevator reached well into the 80s before it finally stopped and we were ushered through a final security check before being allowed out on to the open balcony area at the top. Just beyond the metal detector, I was halted by a call from behind. 'Excuse me, sir? Is this yours?'

I turned and saw a female security officer holding what appeared to be a New Zealand passport. I instinctively patted my jacket pocket and couldn't feel mine there. It must have fallen out while I was taking my jacket off during the security check. 'I think it might be,' I replied.

'It ... doesn't look like you?' Ah, someone had finally noticed.

'Oh, yeah. That would have been about eighty pounds ago,' I smiled sheepishly.

She seemed surprised, and asked for my name, date and place of birth just to make sure. I quickly rattled them all off, and finally she was convinced enough to hand it back over. The pocket zip was kept tightly done up from then on.

The rest of the day passed without incident. The view from the top of the Empire State Building was incredible, with many a photo taken from many an angle. Later we took another stop downtown to catch a photo of the fire station featured in the movie *Ghostbusters*. A pity about all the scaffolding outside, as it was being renovated, but still, at least we can say we were there.

The next day we planned to take a boat tour for the middle of the day when the weather was forecast to be at its best, and spent a few hours just walking the city either side. During the morning we found our way to the USS *Intrepid*, a retired aircraft carrier turned floating naval museum. The boat ride that followed took us up and down the Hudson and East Rivers, passing close by the Statue of Liberty. Then it was more wandering through the city, looking for places to eat and plenty of window shopping. My sister's Fitbit would register over 19,000 steps by day's end.

The food was super-expensive in many places, to no-one's surprise. We had the option of eating at the hotel restaurant but the prices there were outright prohibitive, so instead we visited a nearby diner where I enjoyed a simple salmon salad. Another time we sampled some of the local pizza, which I wrote off as another one of those 'holiday' things. The base wasn't too thick at least. And we found an underground chicken outlet at one point too.

One place that I was most impressed by was somewhere we found by accident. I'd been recommended one particular restaurant ahead of time, but the selection there still seemed a little carby. But the place next door to it had an amazing range of buffet food similar to what I was used to at the lunchtime cafeteria back home, except this place was far bigger. So I loaded up with broccoli and pork, ate what I could there and took the rest back to the hotel later on.

By the last night, I was utterly spent. New York had really taken it out of me by that point. It had been an exciting time to be sure, but equally exhausting for me as well. Every time we walked through Times Square, it felt like I was being swept along by a river of humanity. Never was I more glad that we'd planned our trip the way we had: do all the crazy touristy stuff first, then enjoy some quieter time with our brother's family afterwards.

On the morning of our departure from the city, I remember looking at myself in the bathroom mirror, and tried to decide what I thought of what I was now seeing. I'd stopped shaving at the start of the journey with the intention of evolving a fuller but close-cropped beard, from what had been a goatee for more than a decade. I cast my mind back to the promise I'd made so many years ago, that I would never go clean-shaven again until I was finally happy with my physical self. Was I there yet? I was certainly happier now, no doubt about that, but I decided I still wasn't quite the finished article, so I settled for a trim of the beard as originally planned.

The train ride out of New York began as the simple reverse of our trip in from Philadelphia, only this time the train continued inland past Philly and through more of that beautiful rolling autumnal countryside towards Harrisburg, where our brother would finally pick the two of us up. It was wonderful to see another familiar face again; another little piece of home, yet so far removed from home itself.

Meeting our American nieces in person for the first time was a lot of fun. They were eager to tell us all about their lives, what they'd been doing at school and so on, but they were particularly excited about Halloween, which at this point was just days away. Already there were a couple of pumpkins about the place.

They offered me plenty of Halloween candy on more than one

occasion, which I politely declined each time. I hadn't thought in advance about how to reply to the inevitable question of 'Why not?' but I tried to put it to them as simply as I could. 'I can't eat anything with sugar in it,' I explained, 'because when I do, I get sick.' They understood immediately. If only more grown-ups were as accepting of this as these children were, I thought to myself.

The eating options around the area were interesting. There were a lot of fast food outlets, even out in the countryside. Every few miles in every direction there was a McDonald's and/or Arby's and/or Taco Bell and/or Burger King, often seemingly in the middle of nowhere. I was impressed by Five Guys, who offered bunless burgers, less so by the cheese steaks at one local restaurant which contained as much bread as they did meat. The food at another restaurant in Reading was decent, if a little expensive.

Easily the best place I ate at while staying there, though, was an hour's drive away, at the most massive buffet restaurant I have ever seen and will probably ever see in my life. The prices were good, and the range of food was even better. Were it a little closer to where we were staying, I would have gladly paid to eat there every day. I even enjoyed the bacon there!

I might not have done as much during that second week as I had during the first, but it was exactly what I needed at that point, and the time flew by just as quickly. At least my brother and I got to enjoy one more game of *Twisted Metal 2* together, for old time's sake.

From there my sister and I began the long trek home. Our brother kindly dropped us off at the same hotel in Philly that we spent a night at coming in, and would spend another night there on the way out. It was a sad moment saying goodbye once again, for which even another round of scrambled eggs and turkey sausages for breakfast the following morning this time couldn't quite fully compensate.

We flew back exactly the way we came in. On the leg from Houston to LA, I was squeezed up tightly against the window by another fellow probably about my age or maybe younger, but who was also bigger than I had ever been, spilling freely into the seats either side of his own. I'd always had that fear of upsetting people next to me back in the day whenever I went flying, but this was the first time I'd directly experienced the opposite side of the equation. Like the people I'd observed back at Houston airport on the way in, I felt pity for this guy more than anger. Some discomfort as well, to be sure, but I had my own pillow to help mitigate the worst of it.

That night in LA we stayed at another hotel beside the airport, where the following morning we ordered a room service breakfast after spotting some low-carb options there. Although mine came with bacon instead of the requested sausages, it wasn't too bad, if predictably expensive once again.

It was a long wait at LAX for our return flight to Auckland. Plenty of time for some plane-spotting, which took on an extra special quality later in the day as some flights would take off directly into the setting sun. Having lived along the east coast of the South Island of New Zealand for my entire life, I couldn't recall having ever seen a sunset this large and low on the western horizon before. It was a remarkable sight.

The terminal was also buzzing that evening with the news that the Chicago Cubs had just won baseball's World Series. Many more dedicated followers had been watching the game on whichever TV screen they could find, but their excitement was infectious enough that even people such as myself who didn't really follow the sport couldn't help but absorb some of that happiness. The whole airport just had a really good vibe about it, a wonderful way to wind up the memory of my United States experience.

And yet, there would be one more highlight to top it all off, as I boarded the overnight flight back to Auckland. I found my empty aisle seat next to a family of four, with the mother to my immediate left. 'Oh, thank God,' she exclaimed at my approach. 'I was so afraid I was going to be stuck next to some horrible big fat guy for the whole flight.'

That earned her a long, hearty laugh in response. 'That's really funny,' I chuckled as I sat down beside her. 'More so than you might think.'

Another 24 hours or so later, when I finally arrived home after almost three full weeks away, I took another photo of my feet on the scales. The end result: 87kg. So I'd put on a single kilogram during the entire holiday.

At first I figured that could have been a lot worse, given some of the things that had been put in front of me over the course of my travels. But on the other hand, I'd still been losing about a pound a week prior to going away, so the true difference between what I now weighed, and what I might have weighed had I not gone anywhere, would have been almost 2.5kg. Quite a divergence, when put that way.

It would take me another month or so to reverse that regression, but for the experience of having glimpsed a part of the wider world in person for the first time, having finally seen my brother again and meeting his young family, it was, of course, entirely worth it.

* * *

The invitation came during a family lunch to mark a birthday in November of 2016. It was totally unexpected; I was still settling back down after having just returned from my big trip overseas, less than three weeks earlier.

Many who were there asked me all about the trip, and the simplest way to answer them all was just to hand around my phone, with all of the photos still on it. But one of my aunts had another question for me. Now that I was only a couple of kilos away from goal, would I be interested in accompanying her on a walk along the Kepler Track next Easter?

I was immediately intrigued. Not because I felt I could do it, or because I felt that I couldn't do it, but because I honestly wasn't sure either way. The only previous comparable experience I'd had was that day climb of Little Mount Peel as a youngster, but this would be a bit different from that in a few ways.

The Kepler Track is a roughly circular loop track located on the outskirts of Fiordland National Park, near Te Anau. One half is relatively flat, while the other goes up and over the mountainside itself. Rather than complete the entire loop, the plan for us would be to walk the easier half in, then back out again the way we came. It would be a longer trek than my earlier climb, but hopefully a much easier one. Hopefully.

The decision was still bouncing back and forth in my mind nearly two months later, when I caught up with my cousin the following January. 'So, I hear you're going on a walk?' she enquired knowingly.

'Well, I'm still thinking about it.'

'Oh no, it's definitely happening all right,' she insisted, with a grin.

'Huh.' So word had gotten out. No turning back now. 'Well, okay, I guess it is, then.'

And just like that, it was all on. Suddenly I had to start thinking about how I might prepare for something like this. Yes, the section of the track I'd be walking would be relatively flat, but 24km in each direction still sounded like a pretty long way for someone with my limited experience. Add to that the fact I would need to be carrying my own supplies in and out, and it didn't take long to figure out that this was going to be something I'd have to put some degree of training into beforehand, if I was ever to hope to make the best of the occasion itself.

So, what to do?

The only idea that really came to mind at first was to just keep walking to work and back every day like usual, but putting extra effort into it, making a real power walk out of it each way. I did manage to set some new personal bests, breaking that half-hour mark once or twice on some days when both the weather and the traffic lights were good. But a track walk like this wasn't really meant to be a race, so I had to rethink things some more.

By February I had begun to add things to my backpack, to help me get used to the idea of the extra weight I would be carrying on the day. It started with an extra pair of shoes, but they didn't seem to add too much for objects of their size. After a week or two I switched the shoes out for a couple of books, and then every few days I added another book, over and over until the pack was eventually fully loaded. By the end of the month I was lugging my entire *Song of Ice and Fire* paperback collection by George R.R. Martin, plus a few extras, to work and back every day.

I stuck it out with my bag full of books for another couple of weeks, and even they started to feel lighter after a while. It was pretty exciting to be able to notice some improvement as I went along, since I'd never really consciously stuck with any sort of physical training routine like this before. Whether or not it would turn out to be enough, I could definitely tell that what I was doing was at least going to help, to some extent.

With about three or four weeks to go, word of what I was planning on doing got around work. One colleague mentioned that he'd done the track a couple of times already, and he reckoned I'd blitz it, which was very encouraging to hear. I hoped that he'd be more right than wrong.

Another colleague expressed concern at the food I was planning on taking in. I wanted to stick to low carb as best I could, so in place of the usual scroggin-type mixes of chocolate, raisins and so on, I was thinking bags of grated cheese and macadamia nuts instead. He was worried about my likely energy levels, but I'd read enough Volek and Phinney at this point to understand that my own food choices were likely to be not just adequate, but potentially preferential. Fingers crossed, anyway.

Into April and with less than a fortnight to go, my aunt dropped off the pack that I would be carrying on the walk itself. It was certainly bigger and heavier than my dinky little thing that I had been wearing to work, but of course it had to be, needing to hold three days' worth of food and clothing. I began carrying the larger pack to work, adding yet another book or two's worth of weight for those final few days.

I remember the drive to Te Anau the night before. The weather was cloudy and the night was dark; the headlights shone upon an empty road, but my thoughts were filled with nervous excitement. Whatever was about to happen, this would surely be a weekend to remember.

It was a cool and misty Good Friday morning when my aunt and I got under way from the carpark area at Rainbow Reach, the skies constantly threatening rain but never following through with anything more than the odd spot of drizzle. Considering the forecast for much of the surrounding region for the next couple of days was a bit stormy, we had every reason to be grateful.

We began by crossing a large bridge, hanging a left and running straight into a sign warning us not to go that way because of a slip. Our curiosity got the better of us though, and so we went through for a look anyway. And sure enough, a large section of the track had slumped down a few metres towards the river below, with a few fallen trees randomly criss-crossing the sunken surface.

Later we would be told that we'd completely missed another alternative set of steps that had been hastily dug out just a few bends earlier. But instead, with the genuine belief that our final destination required us to go this way, we decided to clamber our way through and over the slip itself. Thankfully we made it across safely and soon found ourselves properly back on course again, promising to each other that we would take any further such slip signage somewhat more seriously from then on.

After maybe 45 minutes the forest opened up to our right to reveal a small patch of wetland with a short boardwalk leading out to a viewing platform. The most amazing thing about this place was the noise, or more specifically, the complete lack of it. The water was still, the air was calm, no planes overhead, no insects underfoot. The silence was so pronounced that what little birdsong we heard actually echoed around the trees, and I could clearly hear the flapping of wings as one bird flew across in front of us. This was an unexpected pleasure from what was supposed to be just a very long forest walk.

Another hour or so in, we arrived at Moturau Hut and had a short morning tea stopover with the local ranger. As the first hut in from Rainbow Reach, this spot is popular with family day-trippers, enough to stretch the kids' legs for a bit before turning back home. But for us, turning back now was the last thing on our mind.

After following close to the edge of nearby Lake Manapouri for a while, the shoreline fell away as we moved further inland and began to follow the river that lined the length of the valley floor still ahead of us: the Iris Burn. It wasn't always within our sights, but still close enough to remain within earshot for most of the time.

The forest itself would evolve in fits and starts, the track surrounded by ferns, then moss-covered trees of all shapes and sizes, then back to another stretch of ferns again and so on. Some of the muddier sections of the track had been layered with some extra gravel, while a few other patches looked like they were still in need of some. The worst spots were generally board-walked, with some chicken wire overlaid for extra traction.

Most who walk this track do it in the opposite direction to the way we were walking in, so the oncoming traffic was fairly regular, with friendly hellos exchanged maybe every ten minutes or so. At one point we encountered a Romanian lady who had stopped to take a photo, and she reported that my uncle — the ranger we would be staying with — had told his guests the night before to look out for us coming in. We'd been made famous without us even knowing it.

The track had been reasonably gentle to this point, when suddenly it took a wild turn for the vertical. I had been warned about a steeper section near the far end of our walk, but not this part. That thought had me really worried for my lower limbs as they fought to carry the rest of me up a series of zigs and zags. Then with equally little warning, the track began to drop down again, though thankfully not quite so steeply as the climb before.

It was from about here that the bird life began to get interesting. We rounded another left to another small boardwalk bridge and another tramper carefully lowering himself to get a close-up photo of a robin, just in front of him on the bridge. We waited, expecting the robin to take off at any moment, but it was quite content to offer a few poses to both the other tramper and then to us as well. We also took an opportunity here to refill our water bottles for the first time. The creek underneath was flowing gently but clearly, and the water was beautifully cold and fresh to drink.

Lunch at Rocky Point Shelter was a relatively unremarkable point on the journey. Not much more than a couple of picnic tables under a stilted roof built close to the river on fairly sandy ground, and with light drizzle and no wind about, that meant the sandflies were a-buzzin' and a-bitin'. There was a family of mice based in a small set of rocks and logs in front of us as well, no doubt eager to collect whatever crumbs we might leave behind. The joke was on them though: there are no crumbs in bunless burgers.

The next stretch of forest included some larger streams running from right to left down the slopes towards the Iris Burn. In a couple of cases, this meant crossing over bright green steel bridges, which I was told had been assembled off site, then helicoptered into place and held down with rocks at each end. Near one bridge a section of track had been overrun by a recent rockslide, so the track had simply been re-laid over the boulders then back down to the bridge.

Around mid-afternoon and with maybe an hour and a half to go, we got a nice surprise when my uncle turned up to meet us and escort us the rest of the way. (I have to admit that he and I swapped backpacks for a while at this point, as my shoulders were beginning to complain.) From there, the forest peeled back before another open stretch called the Big Slip, named after a ... you guessed it ... big slip, which dammed the valley floor in 1984 before suddenly breaking one day and wiping out a massive section of valley forest. The track itself was still being constructed in those days, so thankfully it wasn't too big a deal to many of us humans at the time.

The last photo opportunity before reaching our destination was the inside of a large tree to our left that had been hollowed out over the years. There were plenty of birds flitting around this area too: fantails, bellbirds, tomtits and riflemen, but all too hyperactive or shy to be easily caught on camera.

Near the end, the track began to climb again as forewarned, but to my relief it actually wasn't as bad as the earlier stretch that I hadn't been told about. Soon we were past that, and then finally the first sign of civilisation since Moturau six hours earlier emerged before us, as the forest parted once again to reveal a small open flat, featuring the Iris Burn Hut.

My first night there was periodically interrupted by various noises from the natives outside. Mostly kea, but I'm sure I heard a kiwi calling at one point in the night as well. The kea's antics continued into the early hours of the morning, taking to anything loose, shiny or rubbery, as is their way. One took a particular liking to the roof spouting, which was finally enough to get me out of bed and start taking photos at about seven in the morning.

Still somewhat feeling the effects of the day before, I was intent on doing rather a lot less this day, but not so little as to be bored. As the last of the visitors departed the main hut, the three of us set to work cleaning up the place, collecting the odd bit of lost property, sweeping the floor, cleaning the surfaces and so on. Then it was off to do a little track work nearby, raking up some loose ferns that were encroaching on the track itself, then laying out a little gravel in places where it was needed.

Our reward came later that afternoon as the sun finally came out, and the three of us took a short 30-minute walk down a side track to the nearby Iris Burn waterfall. This was as far in this direction as we could go; while the valley continued beyond the waterfall for what appeared to be a good distance further, no track existed beyond the waterfall itself. Past this point, there would have been sections of the continuing forest that no human would ever have set foot upon before. I felt like this was as close to the edge of the world as I was ever likely to reach.

After dinner that evening, my uncle suggested my aunt and I park ourselves back out on the track and see if we meet any kiwi in a spot where he knew at least one hung out. We took a single red light between us (white would have only scared them away) and parked outside on the track for a good hour and a half in the fading light. Sadly, aside from kea to our distant left, and morepork to our distant right, the forest remained mostly quiet.

Still, the venture wasn't a total loss as we remembered a nearby glow-worm pit that we'd also been told about, and stopped by there on the way back. That was a pretty special moment; one couldn't help but marvel at the speckled lime green luminescence on the side of the pit wall, just enough for my nearby gloved hand to cast a shadow in the otherwise pitch-black darkness.

The second night passed more smoothly than the first, the kea having granted us a little more of a sleep-in for the following morning, which was appreciated. However, my legs were again feeling stiff as I got up. Not a good sign for the walk back out, but at least there would be compensation in the form of a lighter pack with less food to carry, and a track leaning slightly downhill overall in the outward direction.

The last day — Easter Sunday — dawned gloomy and grey, but dry. I gave myself a few moments on the bench outside to drink in my surroundings for the last time and reflect.

In a sense it felt strange to feel so far away from anywhere, even though I knew the nearest town was only 25 kilometres that-a-way on the other side of the mountain range. I figured it came down to the 7.5 hours it took to reach this spot; that's about as long as a flight from New York to London.

I thought back to my trip to the States the previous year and remembered how physically small it made me feel. Here I felt a different sense of insignificance, this one based on time. This place has existed as it has always been for far longer than I have, and will continue to do so long after I'm gone. And of course I felt thankful to have accomplished so much in the last two years that I could even be here to see it at all.

There was a certain familiarity about the environment as we began the walk back out that morning. Of course I'd been here before, but this time I was moving in a different direction and at a different time of day, so the light helped shine a different perspective on things as well.

Much like the walk in, it remained cloudy for the first couple of hours back through and beyond the Big Slip, but by the time we made it back to Rocky Point for morning tea, it had become brighter. This time instead of sitting at the picnic tables, my aunt and I parked by the edge of the Iris Burn itself, to refill our water bottles once again. I also took this opportunity to send Dad a text that said something like: 'Hi, if you're reading this, then it means I've reached a point in the track on the way out where we're finally getting reception!'

The stiffness in the legs was all but gone by now, and my shoulders still felt fine with the lighter pack, although my ankles were feeling a little swollen, and my knees began to complain for the first time when doing the mid-track up-and-over, particularly on that steep zig-zagging descent. This time we were moving with the flow of traffic so not so many trampers were coming towards us today, but there were one or two that passed us from behind now and then. No worries, each to their own pace. We had plenty of time anyway.

On that basis, we decided we would press on all the way back to Moturau for a late lunch. It was during the hour and a half or so before then that the sun finally broke completely through the clouds and began to selectively shine its way through the overhead tree cover. I found it hard not to stop at every turn to take photos of the rays as they reached the forest floor here and there, the fresh contrasts adding yet another new dimension to my already picturesque surroundings. Still, it was only once we reached the outskirts of Lake Manapouri again that we realised just how blue the sky had become. The day had really brightened up nicely.

Oh, and I saw Dad had replied to my text as well. Neat.

We arrived at Moturau by early afternoon and happily devoured our lunches. These were salad wraps so not 100% ideal, but hey, I'm travelling. If I was to go off plan at all, better to do it later in the trip so that at least I'd be closer to home, were I to react poorly. But my gut behaved itself, or at worst went ignored in favour of my legs, which had earned a good rubbing while we sat.

I had been pretty good with my food to that point, having brought in sausages and eggs, vege soup, a tin of spam and some pre-made bunless burgers. And I'd only needed a few nibbles of the cheese and nuts along the way as well. In fact I'd never felt overly hungry at any point throughout the entire weekend, despite the physical challenges. I certainly needed to be drinking plenty more water than usual, but there was never any shortage of that available along the way at any point.

The final stretch was predictably busy with plenty of day-trippers at this end of the track, but otherwise uneventful. Nearing the end, we ran into the opposite detour sign and this time followed it, finding a slightly safer way downward than clambering over the slip itself once again. Finally at about 3pm, back over the bridge to Rainbow Reach where it all began two-and-a-half days earlier, we were done at last.

My toes were blistered for a couple of days afterwards. A week on, my ankles were still riddled with the remains of heat rash and sandfly bites, and my knees didn't welcome stairs as easily for a while longer either. My poor shoes didn't even survive the experience at all, but they were somewhat worn going into it anyway.

Still, the pain was only temporary, and the shoes could be replaced. Nothing could take away from what I'd achieved that Easter weekend. To think that two years earlier I could barely walk the 2.5km to work, and now — minus 40% of my body weight — I'd just finished walking 50km across three days through one of the most beautiful corners of New Zealand.

As anniversaries go, this one wasn't half bad.

8 THE DREAM

In every block of marble I see a statue as plain as though it stood before me, shaped and perfect in attitude and action. I have only to hew away the rough walls that imprison the lovely apparition to reveal it to the other eyes as mine see it.
—*Michelangelo*[1]

IT WAS ONLY in early 2018 that I wrote about this privately for the first time, but truth be told, this was something I'd been thinking about for much, much longer.

Growing up, I remember a particular episode of *The Simpsons*, where Homer gets really fat and ends up having to work from home. This more or less goes fine for a while until he slacks off as Homer typically does, and a crisis develops at the nuclear power plant which requires that he physically be there in order to fix it. He struggles to make it in time, then accidentally falls into the gas storage tank, but he's saved by his own obesity when his body literally plugs the hole in the tank, and the disaster is averted.

At the end, Mr Burns offers Homer anything he wants as a reward, and after glancing to his family, Homer asks Mr Burns to make him thin again. Burns tries to train Homer's way out of trouble through sit-ups, before deciding it would be simpler for him to just 'pay for the blasted liposuction.' End episode.

I'd heard of this liposuction idea before I'd watched this. Apparently they literally just suck the fat out of you. It sounded simple enough to me. *The Simpsons* certainly made it seem so. Perhaps this was the solution to my problem?

I used to contemplate this while lying in bed at night as a teenager. It fed into this grand idea that I developed for myself in my mind: wouldn't it be great if I could just go to sleep fat and wake up looking normal? For someone in my position, it was the perfect dream. By far the single biggest issue in my life would be gone overnight, just like that.

So great was the extent to which this issue would dominate my thinking, that at times it was hard to imagine any other problem even worth thinking about at all. School, work, friends, hobbies; how much does my success or failure in any of these areas matter at all, if I'm still fat?

Count Rugen perhaps said it best when he spoke to Prince Humperdinck in *The Princess Bride*: 'If you haven't got your health, you haven't got anything.'

At some point I found the details of a clinic in Christchurch that I thought might potentially have been able to help me. I don't recall exactly when, although I was still living at home, so this would have been my mid to late teens. I also don't recall exactly how, as we may or may not have had the internet at home by that point. If not, then I must have gotten the number from the Yellow Pages or something. But I had the number, and I remember holding on to it for a while, wondering whether or not I should make the call.

One thing I knew for certain was that I would only go ahead with it if nobody could find out that I'd done it. The phone number was toll-free, so it wouldn't appear on the bill. So one afternoon I took my chance when nobody else was at home. I took the portable phone into my room and closed the door, as if the walls themselves could hear me. Then I sat down on my bed, and I dialled the number.

A lady answered at the other end and I asked about what the

costs were for liposuction. She asked for where, and I replied: 'Everywhere.'

'That's … not really what liposuction is for. Is there a particular area of the body giving you problems?'

All of it. 'Maybe my tummy?' I offered. It was the biggest of my problems, I supposed.

Her answer was somewhere in the thousands, which was an immediate disappointment, though it did offer some insight as to Mr Burns' generosity to Homer. I pretended that it was still a possibility for the sake of continuing the conversation, to find out more about how it worked anyway.

Apparently it was much like what *The Simpsons* had suggested: they literally just suck the fat out of you. But she also said that the procedure can hurt a lot, and there's a good chance of bruising and/or swelling for a while afterwards as well. Okay, that's 'something I'll have to think about for a bit,' I told her, before thanking her for her help and leaving it there.

Hmmm. Both expensive and painful. The former obviously meant that it wouldn't be happening any time soon, if at all. And even if I was to someday be able to afford it, there would likely be some degree of discomfort both during and after. That temporary discomfort would have to be balanced against the inconvenience, discomfort and shame I already had to deal with every day as a consequence of being fat.

Oh well. No point in making any hard decision about it until I could afford it, anyway. So I parked the idea for the time being, but I never, ever forgot about it.

* * *

After a relatively hectic time in 2015 and 2016 as far as my health was concerned, 2017 was intended to be a year of reflection, of consolidation. By this time I was as happy with my physical self as I'd ever been; 55kg gone from my life, and with any luck, for good.

However, what I came to observe over the course of that year was the legacy of having carried all of that extra weight for so long beforehand. My skin, having been forced to accommodate so much more than it was ever supposed to, had been stretched to its very limits in places. But now all of a sudden, the pressure was off for the first time. Now in places, there was skin that was actually surplus to requirements.

To be fair, most of it was no more than cosmetic. Some of the looseness around my neck, for example, made me look a bit older all of a sudden. There was also a bit extra under my arms and between my thighs, but that could all be hidden away entirely underneath my clothes. By far the worst of it though was my belly. From the button down, I had been left with a distinctively loose roll of skin that I could actually grab and hold with both hands.

I had already read that this could potentially become an issue for some people who lose a lot of weight, but the general consensus had seemed to be that the chances of it all snapping back into place were greater, the younger you were. So I figured that at 39, I should be able to just give it the time it needs to sort itself out.

Perhaps I could also nudge it along with a little bit of exercise. But deep down, I knew that was less likely to happen, beyond the extent to which I was already doing it. Walking to work and back, half an hour each way, five days a week. A few push-ups here, a plank or two there. Was that all not enough? Perhaps it might be for the rest of the extra bits, but for my tummy, not so much.

So it was over the course of 2017 that I first began to seriously consider surgery as an option once again. After a quiet look around online, it seemed to me that I might be looking at either liposuction or possibly a tummy tuck. The two read as being similar, although a tuck is apparently more invasive and can involve a tightening of the abdominal muscles at the same time, if need be.

One of the first things I came to understand about these sorts of procedures was that both the patient and the surgeon ought to be sufficiently convinced that the weight that had been lost wasn't going to come back. After all, what'd be the point in getting something like this done if I was just going to ruin myself again afterwards?

Well, in my case I was feeling pretty confident, as I had already been keeping the weight off now for a number of months. And now that I had figured out what was working for me, I had no reason to deviate, and thus no reason to expect any great rebound for the foreseeable future.

From the surgeon's point of view, I had read that the chances of them agreeing to do the procedure could depend on how long the weight had already been kept off beforehand. In other words, the longer I waited before making contact, the more likely they'd agree to go ahead with it. That sounded fair enough to me.

Without really knowing the best way to find the right surgeon, I decided to ask my doctor about my options in October of that year. He soon offered the name of a surgeon to whom he was prepared to refer me if I wished. Wow, just like that, huh? Well, now that I knew I could get an appointment with someone without too much trouble, and that all I needed to do was to say yes, I found it harder to do so than I'd first imagined. Having had the idea floating around in the back of my mind on and off for over 20 years, the prospect of it suddenly becoming a reality felt like a bit too much, a bit too soon.

So I gave myself the upcoming summer to think about it some more. If I was actually going to get it done, I would hope for a time somewhere in winter, so that my recovery period would be during the time of year when I'd be more likely to spend my time inside anyway, and then hopefully be more or less right again by the following summer. I guessed that that would mean getting things organised during the autumn, and so at the end of that summer in February 2018, I finally went ahead and asked my doctor for that referral.

The card for the appointment at the surgeon's clinic arrived in the mail a couple of weeks later, and at the end of March I went to meet him for the first time.

Like my past visits to the gym, I was a bit nervous going in. The stakes were different this time around, but somehow still felt like just as big a deal to me. First the surgeon would have to agree to offer the procedure. But if he did, then for me to give the go-ahead in return, I'd have to be able to place complete trust of my physical self to that surgeon, who would then literally cut a piece of that self away. It would be a big decision either way.

Soon enough he appeared and ushered me into his office. We sat down and he began asking about my recent history. 'So, I hear you've lost a bit of weight lately?'

'Yeah, something like that,' I smiled, as I gave him the cliff notes from the last three years or so: 55kg gone in 21 months, the last 50 of which came from a low-carb diet across 15 of those months, and which had more or less been kept off in the 15 months since reaching my goal.

'Good job, well done,' he nodded, taking notes along the way. He wasn't overly exuberant about it, but then he didn't need to be; I was proud enough of myself for the both of us. 'So what can I do for you today?'

I told him of the physical legacy of that weight loss, having been left with a little excess skin in a few places, but particularly the lower abdominal area which — unlike the rest of it — was still having a day-to-day impact, still getting in the way of being able to fit shirts properly. 'I don't know exactly whether I'm a suitable candidate for liposuction or a tummy tuck or whatever, but I'm hoping that's something you can possibly help me to figure out?'

'All right, well let's have you hop onto the bed and we'll take a look and see what we're dealing with.' He checked things out, and quickly determined that there was indeed enough excess that could be removed surgically if I wanted it gone. He was also able to detect that my abs had separated a bit over the years as well, so the more suitable procedure for me would in fact be the tummy tuck.

He then went through some of the details of the procedure, answering many of the questions that I had for him without my even needing to ask them.

What happens in the procedure itself? Basically they'd cut the excess roll away, they'd stitch my abs back together while I was open on the table, then sew me up again when done. The belly button underneath would also stay where it is, so in the process of stretching the remaining skin down into place, a new hole would be cut into that skin to accommodate it. I'd be left with a big, long scar across my front from hip to hip, but the stitches themselves would be self-dissolving, so there'd be none to have to remove in the aftermath.

How long does it take? Typically a few hours, for which I'd definitely be knocked right out. It's a pretty major operation, no two ways about it.

How badly does it hurt? Ideally, not that much at all. There would be plenty of pain meds immediately afterwards, but they'd be phased out gradually over the following weeks. The longer-term effects would be some general tightness and some numbness that may linger for months or possibly even years. The effects of the anaesthesia would prevent me from being allowed to drive for at least a few weeks as well.

What's involved in recovery? Lots of rest, but regular light movement such as walking would be ideal to keep the circulation flowing and help prevent clots. Initially there would be a couple of small drains left hanging out of my stomach to handle the excess fluid as the swelling and bruising slowly settled down, but they'd be removed once the need for them subsided.

And of course, what would it all cost? For me, it would amount to a full five figures. I gulped visibly at that news, but the surgeon added some helpful perspective, reminding me that I was still just shy of 40; if all went well, I could live with the benefit of the result for quite some time to come. When spread out over the duration of, say, another 40 years, the cost didn't seem so bad.

Finally came the moment to make the call. I took a deep breath. 'I'm inclined to want to go ahead with it,' I told him, 'but I need to make sure of a few other arrangements first.' This was the truth; I still hadn't told anyone else about the idea yet. If I wasn't able to secure the post-op working and living arrangements, it couldn't happen anyway. And in the meantime, I could make absolutely certain in my own mind that I was truly prepared to go through with it.

The surgery had a waiting time of a few months, which at that time meant that the earliest I could book a date would mean somewhere around the end of June or early July, right at the darkest stages of winter. That sounded pretty good to me.

The first thing to do was to confirm the time off from work. I was a little worried about the possible reaction to the idea of taking an even longer break than I'd done for my trip overseas in 2016, for which some had been a little grumbly. But this time around the support from work was unanimous. I planned to take a clean break from all work for three weeks, then spend another three weeks working part-time from home. That would give me time to wait out the driving stand-down period, as well as time to build up my physical strength to be able to walk all the way in to work once again.

The second thing was to confirm post-surgery hosting arrangements, as the expectation would be that I'd be unable to physically look after myself for a short while afterwards. I had a couple of options available to me, but eventually I settled with a good friend and colleague whose family lived across town.

The third thing was to confirm online grocery shopping options. I did the research and established that of the various supermarkets in town, one of them indeed offered online shopping and home delivery. This was important as, even once I was home, I still wouldn't be allowed to drive for a while longer, so that was another box ticked.

With these obstacles all accounted for, there didn't seem to be any reason left to say no. And so one Tuesday in May, I phoned the clinic to say yes and confirm a surgery date of the 3rd of July. Bam, done. I couldn't help but chuckle at the absurd simplicity of the moment afterwards; I had just committed to a major life decision in much the same way as one might typically commit to a haircut.

From here on, the planning would have to move towards a new level of detail. Across June I began structuring my work in such a way that saw me trying to tie up as many loose ends as possible as the big day drew closer ... only to then have to have the date moved to the 31st of July due to a clash in booking. The anticipation was going to be pretty well drawn out for this one.

While waiting, I remember thinking ahead to a point beyond the surgery, and wondering which size of T-shirts that I might ultimately be able to fit. I ordered the same one online in both L and XL sizes, so I could try them both afterwards, and then look to a new 'final' range once I knew for sure which size would eventually become mine.

Not only did the shirts soon arrive in the mail, but so did the surgery paperwork with about four weeks to go before the revised date. Suddenly I was having to answer some serious questions and hand over some serious money in the form of a deposit. Things felt a whole lot more real at this point; it was only then that I began to feel a little nervous for the first time.

During those final weeks I thought some more about what I would be eating during my recovery. My usual work-based lunch options would be off the table; instead of just being responsible for making my own dinners, I would have to make my own lunches for a while as well. I probably had enough of my own options to cover both, but it would be worth revisiting some past food ideas that I'd previously put aside. Anything I could do to further increase the variety of my meals would be helpful.

By chance, another conversation with my brother on the subject revealed that he had recently started making avocado smoothies. I was still a bit sceptical about the prospective tastes of such a concoction given my previous attempts with avocado, until he mentioned that he sweetened his with stevia. That eventually led me to a local equivalent brand of sugar-free drinking chocolate, which, when tossed into a blender along with some ice cubes and a little cream, actually turned out pretty well.

Another potential new option was identified the day I spotted bags of bacon scraps at the supermarket. I'd never really been into bacon much in the past, but these scraps were small and fairly fatty-looking, so I surmised that perhaps they could serve as an alternative to the chicken that I'd been having with my stir-fry veges. If I got the ratio of meat to veges right, the strength of the bacon flavour wouldn't stand out so much. And once again, this proved to measure up nicely after a couple of attempts.

As the weeks trickled down into days, I registered for home delivery of groceries, and loaded up with extra supplies of nonperishables at the supermarket in advance. The freezer was filled with various meats including the bacon, but the fridge was left mostly empty, as fresh vegetables, eggs and dairy products would form the basis of those first few post-surgery orders once I was back home.

The search for some proper support pillows was a long one, only succeeding with about a week to spare when I picked up a couple of tri-pillows from one local department store for my back, and then finally found a couple of short bolster-style cushions at another store, with which my knees would be able to remain bent while lying in bed during the recovery period.

Thinking ahead, my options for things to do during that recovery period were hard to predict. I presumed I would be spending a lot of time watching TV or listening to the radio. If I had the strength to hold a book, maybe I could do some reading; my work-in-progress at the time was *The Big Fat Surprise* by science journalist Nina Teicholz.[2] Or maybe I could even do some writing of my own, though that might have to wait until I was able to sit up more fully.

Most of the last weekend of July was spent cleaning up the place. I don't enjoy housework any more than anyone else, but I felt it made good sense to attack as much as I could now, while I was still physically able to do it. I couldn't know when I might be able to do any of it again. ''Twas the night before surgery,' I wrote on social media, 'and all through the house, Brendan had cleaned because bugger doing it all afterwards.'

My last supper on the Monday night was a tuna and cheese filled omelette. Later that evening it was off to the hospital for the pre-op appointment. The surgeon asked me about my expectations for the result, and I actually found that quite difficult to answer; I'd been overweight for my entire life until only recently, so I didn't really feel like I had any meaningful frame of reference to go by. 'Just make sure I'm still symmetrical, please?' was about all I could come up with. He predicted I'd be pretty happy with the outcome as far as that was concerned.

Tuesday morning and no breakfast as they wanted an empty

stomach, but I didn't usually have breakfast any more so that was no big deal. The taxi picked me up at 6:30am, I was admitted at 7am — the first on their list for the day — and they mapped out my tummy and began dosing me up at about eight. Everything suddenly felt like it was happening very quickly.

I lay there quietly, trying to stay relaxed, but it was impossible to escape the thought that this moment represented the final realisation of a dream going back more than two decades. My mind flashed all the way back to *The Simpsons*. The actual circumstances here were slightly different as I had in fact lost the weight already, and this was just the clean-up job at the end of the road, the finishing touch to my own weight loss story. But still, here I was, about to go to sleep looking not quite normal ... and about to ... wake up looking ... normal ... er ...?

* * *

You know how usually you'll wake up after a good night's sleep, having recognised at some level that time had passed while you were out? Well, I didn't get that feeling at all after I woke up in a strange room with the clock reading about 1:30pm. More than five hours was missing from my memory, but for all I knew, it had only been five minutes and it was the clock on the wall that was wrong.

I was aware of the presence of at least two people working around me, but had no idea who they were. 'Is it done?' I asked weakly, and somebody said yes. I remember having more questions, but at this point I no longer remember what any of them were. I was lacking the strength to ask any more at the time anyway, and would doze on and off for the rest of the day.

It was suggested to me later that evening that I should have something to eat, but I honestly wasn't hungry at all. I presumed the IV line had something to do with that. When it was removed after it ran out overnight, I was finally ready for something on Wednesday morning. Does IV fluid break a fast? If not, then I'd just incidentally set myself a new personal best of about 36 hours.

Hospital food generally has a mixed reputation, but here there was a good range of low-carb-friendly options; I could just phone for whatever was available from the menu, and I'd have it in front of me in maybe 15 minutes. For each of the three mornings that I was there, I had an omelette filled with cheese and salmon, and I still didn't feel like lunch but for dinner I had a bunless burger one night, and some beef stir-fry on the other.

There was a TV above the bed, which helped pass the time nicely. I didn't sleep very well on the first night, but each night that followed was progressively better. It was annoying to have to be woken up in the night for more pain meds, but I guess it would have been equally annoying to have woken up in the morning in pain.

The surgeon popped in for what he said was his second visit, so I must have been too out of it the first time he passed through, as I didn't remember that at all. He told me that everything had gone well, that the operation went longer than expected but that was because he was also able to remove more than expected: the total amounted to about 1.4kg or three pounds worth of skin and tissue.

My midsection felt super-tight to the touch, but there was no natural feeling in that area whatsoever. I wasn't even able to look down at it at first, no matter how much I wanted to. So I had to settle for the occasional physical examination every now and then, just to remind myself that it was still there, for the most part at least, and to have plenty of patience in the meantime.

I had been warned beforehand to avoid coughing or sneezing if at all possible, as the muscles needed to be given time to rest and heal without the sudden spasms that would occur with each action, and that each such action would hurt quite a lot. But I could feel the need for a cough coming on anyway at one point, so I made sure to wait until a nurse was there, just in case, and ...

... Ow. Yeah, they were definitely right about the pain there. That was one lesson learned the hard way. From then on, I would do my best to try to clear my throat without the need for a full-on cough, where possible.

Learning to climb out of bed again was an interesting experience.

I had to roll onto my side near the edge of the bed with my legs bent into a sitting position, and then push myself upright while keeping my legs bent. I felt so tight around my middle that I couldn't really straighten myself fully, even if I wanted to. As such, it wasn't really possible for me to stand upright either, so my first few attempts at walking again required the aid of a wheeled walking frame. This must be what getting old feels like, I joked to myself.

The two drains below the scar line were doing their part fairly well. One of them was removed on the Thursday and the second one nearly followed soon after, but the drainage picked up on the other side at that point, so that one had to stay in for a while longer yet. When I was discharged to my friend's place on the Friday, I had to carry a small, tightly sealed bottle with me, attached to that remaining drain.

The following Saturday morning I had just enough strength to sit up at a desk for a short while, and returned to my journal for the first time since the surgery. 'The compression garment around my midsection feels uncomfortably tight, sleep tends to happen of its own accord rather than to any schedule, I still can't stand up straight and I still get light-headed just trying to walk around at my own pace,' I wrote. 'This recovery period is the part I know I'm not going to enjoy, but I'm still looking forward to whatever comes beyond that.'

For the first few days of that first week out of hospital, I received daily visits from a nurse to check my remaining drain. Like many of the staff at the hospital itself, she was fascinated by my weight loss story. I supposed that people in her line of work might appreciate a good news story now and then, given the sorts of issues they might otherwise have to deal with every day. So I was happy to show her some before-and-afters.

My host's family, to their credit, were all wonderfully supportive, each in their own way. 'You've shrunk,' his six-year-old daughter once told me. 'I remember when you used to be ...' Her voice trailed off as she paused to consider her next word. '... thicker?' Even their dog was more than content with the company of my simple, largely immobile self during the day while everyone else was at school or work.

My first follow-up appointment with the surgeon was during the middle of that week, to and from which my friend kindly drove me. To my own untrained eyes, the body looked a right old mess at this time: bruised, scarred, swollen, misshapen. But to the eyes of the surgeon and the nurse at his clinic, they were quite impressed. The tape over the scar itself had held on nicely thus far, even through the occasional shower. The pain meds had been doing their job, even though I'd already begun scaling back the dosage slightly, so far without issue.

It was at that follow-up appointment that the second drain was finally removed. That was an eagerly anticipated step in the recovery process, to no longer have to deal with the inconvenience of carrying a bottled drain hanging out of the front of me wherever I went. Not that I could go very far anyway of course, but still, it was something.

I also picked up a second abdominal binder that I could alternate with my first, allowing for each to be washed between uses. This one actually turned out to be a bit bigger and more comfortable than the first one, but I assumed that things were supposed to have been kept fairly tight, so I wore it as tightly as the first one to compensate for its increased size.

As impressed as they were at the appointment, however, they reminded me that I was only just into my second week post-op, and that I still needed to allow myself the full six-week period to properly heal. I definitely still had a long way to go.

Over the course of the week I also took the opportunity to try ordering a few groceries online for the first time. My hosts weren't specifically low carb, so I ordered a few things for myself that were, including a few protein bars that my visiting nurse had suggested I try while I heal. The intention was never to make a permanent habit out of such things, but just to serve as a convenient option for as long as I was still more or less out of action.

I also discovered a brand of peanut butter containing 'high oleic' peanuts, which apparently contained more monounsaturated fat than standard peanuts. There were also some chia seeds mixed into it, which saw me adding a couple of spoonfuls to my morning smoothie across the week, giving them a nice nutty flavour. The only problem with the peanut butter was that it was still one or two more carbs higher than I normally allowed myself, so once again, this was just a temporary thing until I was properly back on my feet.

It felt like it would be a long time before I'd reach that point again. Most of my time that week was spent curled up in bed, as I wasn't capable of much more than that for anything more than a few minutes at a time. The daily shower was quite the ritual at first, typically requiring a good lie down of an hour or more afterwards.

Consequently, I wasn't able to write much in my journal that week at all. I wasn't even able to do much reading either, as I hardly had the strength to hold a book upright, let alone maintain any great degree of concentration for any meaningful period of time. So, like at the hospital, that first week out was spent mostly alternating between TV and sleep.

This was probably the point during my recovery at which I felt my lowest. It was a scary sight to have seen myself unwrapped at the clinic for the first time, and I had felt plagued with feelings of doubt and regret ever since. What had I done to myself? Had I made the right call? Was this all a terrible mistake? And as much as I appreciated the support of my host family, I felt guilty for being the burden that I was. I was glad to finally return to the comfort of my own home the following weekend, to just get out of everyone else's way and keep to myself for a while ...

* * *

Settling into a new routine that first week back at home didn't take too long. One of the first things I did was order the online groceries: mostly veges and dairy, since I had already bought a pile of meat in advance. Their arrival the following morning was straightforward, and with all of that packed away, I felt like I wouldn't have to leave the house again at all for a good while, regardless of whether or not I was capable of doing so.

My next follow-up meeting with the surgeon was on Wednesday

of that week, for which I took a taxi this time, there and back. 'Wow,' I remember thinking to myself, as they politely ferried me either way across town. 'These guys are really good drivers.' It wasn't until much later that I realised it was more the fact that my own senses were still so dulled from the lingering effects of the anaesthesia following the surgery that made their skills stand out in my mind, that they could spot and react to approaching traffic from every direction so quickly. They really weren't kidding when they'd warned me not to drive myself, and I was glad that I'd paid heed to that advice.

Between rides, the appointment itself went fine. For the most part, everything seemed to be progressing according to plan. A few more surrounding bandages came off, but the main tape covering the scar itself remained on, and was supposed to do so for as long as it could. The bruising, which had looked really nasty in some places earlier, was also now beginning to subside, which I was relieved to see.

Most of that first week at home alone was once again spent watching TV. I was actually finding a lot of those low-key home and garden type shows quite good for dozing off to while lying in the recliner at nights, as a variation on the bed full of tri-pillows and cushions.

My strength was beginning to recover, but still only slowly. I could now manage to lift a basket full of wet laundry again, at least. 'I won't lie, it has been frustrating at times,' I wrote in my journal, 'but I try and take the day-by-day view that if I could survive being fat for 30+ years, I can survive these few weeks/months of recovery, if it means another 30+ years of being how I want to be.'

That weekend I dared to take a couple of short walks from home halfway down the hill and back for the first time, just to see if I could manage. I was definitely a lot slower, still not quite able to stand fully straight, and wasn't sure about my endurance for the eventual return to work full-time in a couple of weeks, at which point I would need to be able to walk 2.5km in a single stretch. Still, I remembered that there were a number of park benches scattered across the middle of town, each of which I could use as rest stops if I still needed them by then.

The following week was the last week of August, during which I tried doing a little work again for the first time since the surgery. Just a few hours from home each day, and they were mostly spread across the day, as I still felt the need for regular breaks. Even almost a month post-op, my brain was still clearly in need of more time to fully get back up to speed.

Progress, though, continued to track steadily. At my next follow-up appointment with the surgeon, he reckoned I was healing up fairly well for six weeks. When I pointed out to him that it had actually been only four weeks, he was amazed; he wasn't sure he'd seen anyone heal from something like this so quickly before. He told me I was good to drive now, so I went for a cruise up and down the nearby motorway just to get a feel for it again, and overall it felt pretty good. 'The side streets are still a bit of a challenge, as I still feel it when turning my body to look both ways at intersections,' I wrote, 'but I'm sure that will improve with time.'

By this time I had also noticed that both of my abdominal binders were beginning to fit me more easily than before, the overlap now extending by maybe a couple of inches or so. The initial swelling was beginning to subside at last.

Once I'd realised that, I decided it was worth trying on those two T-shirts that I'd ordered prior to the surgery, to see how they would fit me now. To my delight, the L was now a nice comfortable fit all over, so I swiftly ordered a new round of L-sized tees for the upcoming summer. The leftover XL I gave to my friend who looked after me in that first week out of hospital.

The sleeping continued to improve. Through most of August I had retained most of my original pillow setup, but if I woke in the night, I would experiment with a few hours minus a pillow here or there, just to give myself the freedom to spend a short while now and then in different sleeping positions, beyond simply being on my back all the time. To be able to catch just an hour or two on my sides — knees still slightly bent of course — was a very welcome change.

The pillow arrangement continued to simplify into September, by which time I was finally able to do away with both tri-pillows entirely. This finally freed me up for a lot more time on my sides, but my knees still had to remain bent for a while, and I was still a long way from being able to sleep on my front.

By now I was also walking up and down the hill from home every day, building up my strength for the upcoming return to work. A couple of times I even ventured part of the way into town, and while I certainly wasn't going to be breaking any speed records any time soon, and I did need to stop at the occasional park bench for a rest now and then, it still felt really good to get out and about to the extent that I could, once again.

I was able to drive myself to my next follow-up appointment. Until now, I'd always been told that the original tape needed to stay on the wound for as long as it was able to, but generally the expectation was that it would only last for a few weeks. Well over a month later now, however, mine was still comfortably hanging on, so they finally decided it was time to remove it anyway.

Looking through the tape before it had come off, I could see a dark stripe through it that, in places, looked up to a quarter inch thick. I'd assumed that was the underlying scar having widened over time, and in comparison with other examples I'd seen in online videos, I thought mine didn't look too great when viewed through the tape.

But the difference once the tape came off was amazing. It turned out that the thick dark stripe I had seen beforehand was just the result of old blood that had seeped through the wound in the first few days following the operation. But underneath all that, the actual scar itself looked almost as thin as if I'd drawn a line of red pen on myself. It was soon redressed with some thinner tape, and came with instructions that when this lot would be ready to come off of its own accord, that too would be that.

They also told me that I didn't need to be wearing my binder any more, but by this time I'd actually developed a strange sense of security around wearing it. Still, it wasn't quite as comfortable wearing it while sitting down as it was while standing or lying straight, so that was my opening towards a sort of transition process to wean myself off it altogether.

In fact, they decided I looked so good at this point that I didn't need to come back for any further follow-ups at all. This appointment would turn out to be my last. The worst was now over. 'So I am now officially no longer a tummy tuck patient,' I wrote the following weekend. 'While I personally feel like I'm still maybe only about 80% recovered, as far as both the hospital and the clinic are concerned, I'm home and I'm free.'

But by far the greatest thing was just being able to tuck a shirt in and see my belt without having to find a place for that extra skin any more. For a goal that had seemed so simple on the face of it, being finally able to achieve it for the first time in my life meant even more to me now than I had previously expected. It was hard to keep the emotions in check that night.

There were still other things that I could have had touched up if I'd wanted to, of course. My neck, my arms, my thighs. The surgeon himself had made the offer, but I'd said no thank you. Those other bits and pieces, they still had their place as they were. They can be my battle scars, the things I can show people who don't believe me when I tell them that I used to be fat.

But now? Now I finally felt ... normal. To external eyes I might have looked normal enough already, but only now did I actually *feel* it. It was all that I had ever hoped for, and it was all that I had dreamed it could ever be. It had been a fair ordeal to reach this point, but I could not have been happier with the end result. I could not have been happier with everything.

On Monday the 10th of September 2018, six weeks after the surgery and shortly before my 40th birthday, I made my return to the office full-time, ready to resume my work there properly after three weeks of chipping away part-time from home. I'd made it there all the way in one go too, without having to make any extra rest stops at all.

And for the first time in almost two decades, I was clean-shaven.

9 THE KITCHEN

Sugar, sweets of all kinds, potatoes in every form I forbid unconditionally.
The quantity of bread is limited at most to 3 to 3½ oz a day, and of
vegetables I allow asparagus, spinach, the various kinds of cabbage and
especially the leguminous. ... Of meats I exclude none, and the fat in the
flesh I do not wish to be avoided, but on the contrary sought after. I permit
bacon fat, fat roast pork and mutton, kidney fat, and when no other fat is
at hand I recommend marrow to be added to the soups.
   —*Dr Wilhelm Ebstein,* Corpulence and its Treatment, *1884*[1]

HISTORICALLY, I'd never really been fond of the kitchen. It was, after
all, the place where all those evil calories came from, the calories that
I was always told were making me fat. When growing up, the most I
ever did in there was to prepare my breakfast and make everybody's
sandwiches for school lunches in the mornings, and wash or dry the
dishes at night.

It took me a while to grow accustomed to the idea of spending
any meaningful amount of time in that part of the house again after
actively avoiding it for so long, but I'm so glad to have since gotten
used to that transition, at least to the point where I feel I can more or
less get by.

Once I'd finally gotten over that initial mental hurdle of simply coming to terms with LCHF as a viable proposition at all, the next big challenge for me was going to be working out the details behind how to follow it. I'd settled on my personal rules for the general concept — never go hungry, keep the carb count as low as possible while still preserving sufficient variety, and track my progress — but I still had to work out the specifics of exactly what sorts of food I could eat.

Identifying low-fat food is easy: these days it generally tells you that on the front of the packaging already. But for a while there I didn't really have any internal instinct for what sorts of food might be low in carbs at all. It was just such a foreign idea from the start.

That made the early months of my diet fairly repetitive as I had kept to the same few dishes for the sake of sticking to my rules. But over time as I kept reading and researching, more and more options began to emerge from every different direction: books, websites, friends and family and so on.

Eventually I found myself planning my diet like I might plan the development of a character of mine in a video game. I hadn't realised it at first, but once I recognised the parallels, I found this to be a really compelling way for me to think about it. It was like planning a strategy for perhaps the most incredible game of all: the game of personal health, the goal being not just to attain it, but to then keep it afterwards as well.

In gaming, the art of working out the best possible gear combination for your character is called 'min-maxing'. You identify the less desirable traits versus the more desirable ones, and then set out to minimise the bad ones and maximise the good.

Take a character in some fantasy role-playing game, for example. You want the weapons that do the most damage to your opponents, and you want the strongest armour to provide the best possible defence against incoming damage. Individual weapons and armour pieces might not always be the best items on their own, but when combined they come together to provide an optimal statistical combination for success.

It's not always that simple though. Some items might have several sets of statistics that present some kind of trade-off between them, so that no one item in the game is considered the best universally, but might be the best for a certain playstyle only. For example, the armour with the best defensive stats might also be the heaviest, and that may impact your character's performance in other ways, like not being able to move as fast or carry as much loot. These compromises might be acceptable if you're working on some oafish barbarian-type character, but for a stealthy thief the 'best' armour might be something completely different.

All of these principles can apply to nutrition as well. We can break down and identify a perceived value for each of the various macronutrient groups according to the general principles of any given dietary approach. When I came to try to figure out LCHF in this way, I eventually settled on the following profile of macronutrient priorities, based on what I had learned. In this process I was guided by the principle of Occam's razor, once paraphrased by Albert Einstein to the effect of 'everything should be made as simple as possible, but not simpler,'[2] so as not to lose sight of some important details:

- **Carbohydrates** = bad, fibre less so.
- **Protein** = good, complete sources preferred.
- **Fat** = depends on the type:
▷ *Good fats* = monounsaturated, saturated and omega-3 polyunsaturated fats.
▷ *Not so good fats* = omega-6 polyunsaturated fats; avoid in large quantities.
▷ *Bad fats* = trans fats.

Now that I'd worked out what I wanted to minimise and what I wanted to maximise, I could then start to figure out what sorts of foods were going to fit this profile. Suddenly I was starting to appreciate the discovery of a suitable food option, in much the same way that I would get excited at finding a quality piece of gear in a game: it all came down to the numbers, and understanding which of those numbers meant more than others.

And where would one find these numbers? More often than not, on the food labels; or, where the product did not come with a label — such as fruit or vegetables — from a simple internet search.

The standards for New Zealand's food labels, formally known as Nutrition Information Panels, are developed by a statutory authority called Food Standards Australia New Zealand,[3] and whose standards are enforced in this country by the Ministry for Primary Industries.[4] While not perfect, our labels do measure up reasonably well relative to equivalent labelling in other parts of the world, for one important reason: the column listing the nutrient amounts per 100g of food.

Other information was less useful, in my estimation. Information relating to percentages of recommended dietary intakes were of no use, as anything based on existing guidelines had generally been for me up to this point. And numbers based on serving sizes weren't very practical either, as serving sizes could vary wildly from product to product. But a consistent column of numbers per 100g provided the ideal means with which I could objectively compare any two products.

With this information, I was able to take LCHF very literally. First, I set myself an upper limit of no more than 10g of carbs per 100g, later reducing that limit down to 5g once I had built sufficient variety into my diet. Learning to embrace fat again took a little longer, and in some cases required a bit of online research where the types of fats weren't always shown on the labels themselves. But cutting the carbs came first.

Applying this logic, it would soon become clear which sorts of foods were to be avoided. Take wholegrain bread, for example: commonly lauded for its fibre content, but there was also way too much starchy carbohydrate on the label for it to be worthwhile for me. I could always look to green vegetables for more fibre, with far less of the starchy trade-off.[5]

Other foods meanwhile, such as eggs, would emerge as being an ideal fit by the numbers. The challenge in that particular example for me, as someone who traditionally didn't like eggs, would be more about finding a way to work them into the diet to be able to actually enjoy them.

There wouldn't necessarily be many individual foods that would fit all of my macronutrient criteria perfectly, but that was okay, as I wanted to enjoy a decent variety of meals anyway. As long as everything I was eating was steering me in the right direction overall, so that the diet as a whole would still fit the profile as a whole, then that would be fine.

If I were to make compromises, it would have to be for a good reason. One such compromise that I made early on was with tomato sauce; the variety with the least carbs that I could find was 16g/100g, but I still allowed it as I only needed a little bit of it to enable me to enjoy my homemade bunless burgers, so much more than without it. And since there are so few carbs in the other ingredients, the total carb count of the meal would still be fairly low anyway.

All of these rules and restrictions might perhaps come across as a bit imposing to some, but for me, I felt up to the challenge. And as the saying goes: art thrives on restrictions.

* * *

Now armed with some idea of what to do, I was next faced with the dilemma of just how to do it, and what tools I might need in order to be able to do it.

One of the habits that I was able to form very early on was the concept of a shopping list. This was important especially at first, as my diet was changing so radically that I felt compelled to be writing everything down just so I could remember it all. As I wandered the aisles checking the various food labels, I would also make a note of any new discoveries that I could learn to work with going forward.

In my case, the shopping list concept doubled as a loose kind of food diary as well. The idea of writing down exactly what I was eating each day didn't appeal to me at all, but I eventually realised that by keeping my shopping lists as I wrote them, I was essentially doing that already, even if it was in more of a general sense. These kinds of records weren't necessarily reflective of any particular day's worth of eating, but I've found them to be good enough overall for the bigger picture.

The question of what utensils and implements I would need in my kitchen was just something I figured out for myself, as meal options began to emerge from wherever they would. Once I'd decided on a certain meal idea based on the things that I was bringing home from the shops, my next step was to work out what I would need in order to prepare that meal.

Some things I already had and was already used to using on a semi-regular basis. Simple things like glasses, dinner plates and cutlery, and of course the microwave. My cheese grater and can opener are both well-worn, but continue to somehow hold together. I've been through a good number of cheese slicers over the years as well.

Some things I already had but I hadn't always been making regular use of them in the past. The stove itself, a few pots, a cutting board and a couple of sharp knives, a wooden spoon, a stainless-steel spatula, an egg beater, a whisk, an ice cube tray.

Then there were things that I didn't have at all, some of which continue to amaze me to this day that I had previously gone without them for so long. Top of this list, would you believe, was a non-stick fry-pan? I use mine a few times a week nowadays, along with a non-stick spatula. I never owned a blender either, until 2018. A full-blown food processor would be useful as well, although I personally settled for a handheld vegetable masher instead. And don't forget the spiraliser, for making noodles out of your vegetables, too.

Many of my meals, as you will discover, are basically some combination of meat and vegetables. And I can understand if that may sound a bit boring to some, at first. A friend once asked me: 'What do you do for filler, like in place of rice for example?'

'Just more of everything else,' I replied. It's the 'everything else' that's more tasty anyway, when you think about it. Imagine rice without curry, spaghetti without sauce, pizza without toppings, sandwiches without fillings, cereal without fruit or milk. On their own, they're all just bland, beige/white, tasteless filler.

Different types of meat and vegetables, on the other hand, are full of flavour, and any of them can be used to build meals of different combinations, all prepared and seasoned in different ways. I've learned that it's possible to make meals that both look and taste quite different from each other, even with some ingredients being reused on more than a few occasions. There's more than one way to consider how to build variety into your diet.

As a still relative newbie to all of this myself, I'm also not a fan of complexity. There's no shortage of recipes out there with lists of 15 or more different ingredients, and many of those ingredients can be hard to find, expensive to buy, or both. Things are kept pretty basic here; I'm assuming that the reader is as green to the kitchen environment in general as I still am. Even now I still find myself sometimes forgetting to get the meat out of the freezer in the morning before work, to defrost across the day!

Most of what I eat is just based on everyday groceries that one can collect from the supermarket. While a couple of things are still on the expensive side (why hello there, salmon; how's it going, steak?), I personally find them worthwhile for the variety that they bring to the diet, both in terms of taste and nutritional value. You could try to live off just the same couple of meals every day if you wanted, but I don't know that I would necessarily call that a well-formulated diet, and I'd probably just find that boring anyway.

Ensuring a certain quality of food can also mean that eating low carb might work out to be more expensive than a more 'standard' diet on a per meal basis. But I've found low carb to be far more satiating overall, to the point where I'm having fewer meals now than I was before, so the cost does tend to work out roughly the same over time for me anyway. Not to mention the prospect of future cost savings for one's own health care on top of that.

One thing I will concede is the added time requirements for preparing low-carb food, compared to living off processed food. But then, I suppose the same would be true of any diet compared to processed food. In fact, looking back, that's probably a key factor behind why I drifted towards so much processed food in the first place, to save ~~dishes~~ time.

Eventually I came around to the idea of spending more time in the kitchen by thinking of it as time spent investing in myself. And as soon as that investment started to pay dividends on the scales after just a few weeks, it was clear to me that the choice was going to be worthwhile.

All of the meals in this chapter form part of my own personal eating plan, and as such they all serve one, although I guess there's nothing to stop you from using bigger pots/pans/trays and upping your ingredients accordingly. Some meals will also result in more dishes than others, though most are manageable enough for me personally that I'm not exactly filling the sink every night.

Refer to the appendices for my complete shopping list, and tables of my complete meal plan, both what I was eating while I was losing weight in 2016 and what I have eaten for maintenance.

* * *

Bunless burgers

This was the very first low-carb meal that I ever consciously prepared for myself. It was lunchtime one weekend in October 2015. For all I knew at the time, this was just going to be a one-off experiment. I was still a long way from being convinced that this low-carb business was actually going to do the trick.

Of the few meal options I had worked out for myself at this point, I figured that this was going to be the yummiest. For that reason, I settled on this as my regular Monday dinner; finally, a reason to look forward to Mondays! And whatever the outcome of this plan, I at least wanted to enjoy it as much as I could along the way.

It turned out to be a pretty good start.

- 2–4 beef burger patties (depending on size)
- a couple of small mushrooms (optional)
- a few leaves of lettuce
- low-sugar tomato sauce or paste
- a few slices of cheese

Place the burger patties in an oven tray and fan bake at around half heat (150°C). Check the oven once you start to hear the patties sizzling; this could be around 15–20 minutes or so, depending on the size and thickness of the patties. Once the tops of the patties have mostly browned, flip them over, and place a few slices of mushroom, if using, on top of each of patty, then leave them to cook for another 10 minutes or so.

When done, remove the tray from the oven and let everything cool for a few more minutes. If you start wrapping them in lettuce too quickly, the lettuce itself can start to cook with the residual heat and go soft.

Peel off a nice big leaf of green lettuce and place your first patty on top. Add a squirt of low-sugar tomato sauce, then a slice or two of cheese. If the lettuce leaf is big enough to fold over on top then do so, otherwise add a second separate leaf to the top. Serve and eat any way you like.

Cheesy scrambled egg with sausages

It was Prof Noakes who stated during one of his presentations in the online course I took, that eggs were among the most nutritious foods that we as human beings can eat, and that we'd all be so much better off if we just had a couple of eggs for breakfast instead of cereal, toast or whatever else it was that we were all otherwise used to.

There was just one problem: I hated eggs.

However, the Prof's case was so persuasive that I decided I just had to find a way to tolerate them. So I gave my brother a call and asked him for ideas, since I knew he had always loved eggs. His simplest suggestion led to what would become my early breakfast staple.

- 2 eggs
- a shot of cream
- some grated cheese
- seasonings to taste
- 1 large or 2 small pre-cooked sausages

Crack the eggs into a microwave-safe bowl, add the cream and beat with a whisk. Grate some cheese into the mixture; the exact amount is up to you, but I give it plenty. Toss the cheese and egg mixture a little with a fork to make sure the cheese is spread around the bowl fairly evenly.

Place the bowl in the microwave and cook on High for about 3 minutes depending on the strength of your microwave, stopping every minute or so to stir the mixture, as the edges will cook faster. When done, take out and add your choice of seasonings and loosely stir into the cooked egg.

Next, put the sausages into the microwave (you may wish to chop the ends off the sausages first if the skin is annoying) and cook them on High for 30 to 60 seconds as needed, depending on their size. When done, cut into small bite-sized chunks and sprinkle them over the eggs in the bowl.

Cheesy filled omelettes

Omelettes are a pretty simple idea. I'd personally always ignored them for most of my life because of the whole don't-like-eggs thing. But what I soon learned from an online recipe video is that you can fill an omelette with all sorts of things, typically cheese and whatever else you like. My brother later also verified this when I checked with him.

I tried a variety of ideas for my omelette fillings in the first few months, including chopped spam, mushrooms, cherry tomatoes, bits of sausage and bacon. But over time, my personal favourite option became grated cheese with canned tuna.

If you've got the time to make one of these for breakfast, then go for it. You might need two of them for lunch or dinner, however, depending on how hungry you are.

- 1 tbsp butter/cooking fat of choice
- 2 eggs
- a shot of cream
- salt/pepper/garlic powder to taste
- ½ can of tuna, packed in olive oil
- some grated cheese

Add the butter to a frying pan and turn up to just over 2/6. Crack the eggs into a bowl, add the cream, salt/pepper/garlic powder and beat with a whisk. Once the butter has melted, pour in the egg mixture and tilt the fry-pan as needed to ensure a fairly even spread.

While the egg is cooking, put half a can of tuna into the same bowl and cut up loosely with a knife, before grating some cheese over the top. Toss the cheese and tuna mixture by hand until it's all mixed in reasonably well.

Carefully scatter the cheese and tuna mixture onto one half of the egg base still cooking in the fry-pan. You'll probably want to wash your hands again at this point once the bowl is empty. The cheese in the pan will slowly melt for the next couple of minutes.

Once you can see the very edges of the egg mixture turning brown, it's time to flip the empty side of the omelette over on top of the filled side. This is easier than it sounds; just remember to use a non-stick spatula if you're also using a non-stick fry-pan, so that you don't scratch the surface of the pan.

Turn the heat back down to 1/6 and let the whole thing just cook lightly for a few minutes longer. When ready, the omelette should comfortably slide out of the pan (with a bit of nudging with the spatula if necessary) onto a plate.

Lazy courgetti bolognese with sour cream

This meal has evolved a fair bit since I first started making it. Originally I would prepare the 'spaghetti' separately and then layer the rest on top, but then laziness took hold and now I just throw everything into the one pot instead.

I also used to apply tomato sauce but later switched to canned tomatoes, to further save on carbs. Canned tomatoes are really cheap too, sometimes going for as little as $2 per can when on special.

Finally, I began topping with cottage cheese but at some point switched to sour cream for the increased fat content. You could also use regular grated cheese if you like, but with cheese in three other meals already, I figure it's nice to try to mix things up a little where possible.

- 250g mince
- 2 chicken livers (optional)
- 1 courgette/zucchini
- 2–4 mushrooms, depending on size
- ½ can of tomatoes or some tomato paste
- beef stock to taste
- 60–80g sour cream

Place the mince into a medium-sized pot, flatten the inner surface with it and turn the stove up to around 2/6. If including liver, chop it up and mix it into the mince as well. Turn it over after a few minutes once browned.

Spiralise the courgette and then add it into the pot on top of the browning mince. Now is a good time to slice up the mushrooms, any way you like. After a few more minutes, start 'chopping' the mince and courgette noodles in the pot with a wooden spoon, to the point where you can start to mix the two together. It may seem a bit dry, depending on how long the mince has been cooking, but it won't stay that way for long.

Next, add the canned tomatoes to the pot along with the

mushrooms, and then stir the entire mixture with the wooden spoon. The whole thing should soon start to simmer; just let it, stirring it every other minute or so just to help prevent too much from sticking to the bottom.

Add a few sprinkles of beef stock to the pot between stirs. How much is up to you, just try to avoid shaking it directly into the pot from the container; the steam coming from the pot will get into the stock and make it lumpy. Try just collecting a pinch or two on your fingers, or use a teaspoon if you don't want to risk a mess.

I give the mince a good 20 minutes or more in the pot from start to finish before draining away any excess water and serving on a plate as is, with a healthy dollop of sour cream on top for good measure.

Chocolate avocado smoothie

I struggled with avocados for a long time. I'd always heard right from the start about how awesome they were, but I really didn't like the taste of them at all. On their own I still don't like them now.

Once again it was my brother who eventually came to the rescue for me with this. His suggestion was to use them as a base for making smoothies, and then add whatever sugar-free sweeteners or flavourings I could find to disguise the taste of the avocados themselves.

I wasn't sure about this idea at first. Smoothies seem like a really trendy, even overrated way of eating food these days. But for the sake of finding a way to incorporate avocado into my diet, I bought a blender from the local department store during a sale over Easter 2018, and came up with the following recipe for myself. (A high-powered blender is best for crushing ice cubes.)

- 1 full tray's worth of ice cubes
- 2 large or 3 medium-sized ripe avocados
- 2 heaped tbsp sugar-free drinking chocolate
- 1 tbsp chia seeds or a handful of berries (optional)
- 1 tsp vanilla extract
- 60–80ml cream

First crush the ice cubes in the blender, then slice open the avocados and remove the stones. Once the ice has been crushed, scoop out the insides of the avocados and add them into the blender. Cut the pieces of flesh up with your spoon if need be, and loosely mix the avocado flesh into the ice just so that the blender doesn't have to do all the work.

Next, add the drinking chocolate (and chia seeds or berries if using), then the vanilla extract, and finally the cream. Try to catch as much of the dry ingredients as possible when pouring in the cream, and then stir in what remains of the chocolate powder, otherwise the powder may puff up around the sides of the blender when it starts.

Start the blender on a low setting at first for just a few seconds, then crank it up to whatever smoothie settings your blender supports, and leave it there for as long as it needs, anywhere from 30 seconds to a minute or so.

Serve and eat as you like. My smoothies come out quite thick, my blender is quite large and I'm quite lazy, so I might eat it with a spoon straight out of the blender jug, or possibly pour half into a plate for a dessert-style option for another time. It may not look like much of a feed, but I've found this to be surprisingly filling, sometimes enough to constitute an entire meal on its own.

Fried salmon and spinach with aioli

This was another early concoction that I originally adapted from a recipe book somewhere, but even by then I had learned that salmon stood out as a good source of omega-3 fats, and spinach was consistently appearing near the top of most lists online, whenever I went looking for vegetables considered both the lowest in carbs and the most nutrient dense. The addition of aioli came later and really sealed the deal for me.

Over time this would become my regular Wednesday or Thursday meal, to keep separate from the tuna that I would have in my omelettes on the weekends. It also became one of my more reliable 'whoosh' triggers, a meal that, more often than not, would typically result in my having lost a little weight the next morning.

- olive oil
- 200g salmon fillet
- 1 handful of spinach leaves
- salt/pepper to taste
- aioli to taste

Heat up a fry-pan with olive oil at just over 2/6 and add the salmon fillet. I like to cook it skin side down first as that surface tends to be flatter. Chop up a small handful of spinach leaves while the salmon is cooking.

Once the salmon is becoming noticeably more pale around the edges, it's time to flip it over. Give it at least five more minutes on this side, then I tend to go back for a few more minutes on the original side as well.

When ready, remove the salmon and add the spinach into the pan and just fry it in the remaining oil. This won't take long, no more than a few minutes. While the spinach is frying, remove the skin from the salmon and season with salt and pepper on both sides.

The spinach in the pan will quickly wilt and turn a crispy brown, at which point it will be ready to serve alongside the salmon, plus a good dollop of aioli on the side.

Stir-fry vegetables with chicken or bacon

Vegetables were one of those things that, growing up, I'd always found really bland and unsatisfying to eat. Until, of course, the day I discovered how well they went with tomato sauce, but we can't really go there any more, now can we?

Still, the idea of mixing them up with other flavours stuck with me. When I was young, our vegetables tended to be boiled rather than fried, but I do remember enjoying the differences in both taste and texture when they were fried, and so this idea was my attempt to revisit and further explore that earlier concept.

For the first couple of years the meat accompaniment here was chicken, but later I successfully experimented with using bacon scraps as well, and these days I tend to alternate between the two, or just whatever I feel like on the day.

- olive oil
- 1 small to mid-sized chicken breast or 2 small chicken thighs, or 250g bacon scraps
- 150–250g or 1/4 bag frozen stir-fry vegetables
- 2–4 mushrooms, depending on size (optional)
- soy sauce
- garlic powder/pepper/salt to taste

Heat a fry-pan up to about 2/6 with olive oil and if using chicken, chop the meat into bite-sized chunks. Spread the meat around the pan and let it cook for a few minutes. If using chicken, the chunks will probably each need flipping once or twice to ensure that they are cooked on all sides. The bacon scraps, on the other hand, can just be stirred all together every now and then.

After 5–10 minutes, remove the meat and let stand on a separate plate for a while. Top up the olive oil in the pan if necessary and turn up to 4/6, and now add the frozen stir-fry vegetables, stirring regularly with a wooden spoon so that nothing gets overly burned on any one side.

If using mushrooms, chop and add them to the pan after the other frozen veges are in the pan; the frozens will need a few extra minutes in the pan anyway, while the mushrooms will be fresh.

Stir the veges every minute or so for several minutes until most of them show signs of browning, then turn the heat back down to 2/6 and add the meat back into the pan for another go, this time with the veges.

Add a shake or two of soy sauce, and stir in while everything simmers for a few minutes longer. The sauce should darken the look of everything in the pan once it's stirred in, particularly the meat if you're using chicken. Some garlic powder wouldn't go astray at this point either, again if you're using chicken.

Serve the whole thing on a plate and season with pepper and/or salt, though the salt may not be necessary if using bacon as it has a naturally salty flavour anyway.

Steak and mushrooms with cauli mash

This meal is entirely of my own design, and for the most part consists of a variety of ingredients that I simply couldn't figure out how to prepare in any other way, so they ended up being lumped together into a dinner option of their own.

Steak was always going to find its way into the system at some point, and I recall mushrooms going with it fairly well, at least according to my old pie habit, anyway. And of course the cauli mash serves as the classic alternative to potato.

For the most part I think it works fairly well, and for a couple of years it was my year-round Friday evening meal. These days its status is relegated to winters only, or at least when avocados aren't in season and my smoothies aren't currently an option.

- 250g steak
- a little beef stock
- ¼ of a large head of cauliflower
- 4–6 mushrooms, depending on size
- 1 tbsp butter
- some grated cheese
- salt/pepper/garlic powder to taste

The steak takes the longest to cook, so I start that first with the meat in an oven tray, and a sprinkle of beef stock on top. Start the oven fan-baking at around 150–200°C.

With that under way, break apart the cauliflower into small florets by hand and place into a large bowl half-filled with water. Cover the bowl and microwave on High for about 5 minutes. When done, remove the bowl from the microwave and break up the cauli florets further with the masher, keeping the water there as well, then cover and return to the microwave for another 5 minutes on High.

While that's going, remove the steak from the oven and flip over, adding another sprinkle of beef stock on top before returning to the oven for a while longer.

Slice the mushrooms while waiting, and when the cauli is done a second time, remove from the microwave, drain the water and let stand for a minute. Now is when I add the mushrooms to the steak in the oven; they won't need long.

Add the butter to the cauli and let it melt into the cauli while mashing it. Then add the grated cheese, mash some more, and finally mash in your choice of seasonings. Serve on a plate with the steak and mushrooms once they're also ready.

Meat and vegetable soup

Soup is one of those classic options that works particularly well in the winter, and I saw this as another way of getting my vegetable intake up.

In recent years I've observed that I tend to actually put on a little weight after this particular meal, to the point where I now have it less often than before. I suspect that this happens because even though this is still fairly low in carbs per 100g, there is even less protein and fat per 100g, so in terms of a percentage of total energy, carbs still make up a large proportion of what's there.

My way of attempting to at least partly compensate for this was to add the meat and cheese to it, and I have to say it certainly makes it more enjoyable to eat, but not enough to keep around as a regular

option any more. Its value to me these days is more as a backup
option for when time is short, since this is very quick and easy to
prepare.

- 1 can of country vegetable soup
- ½ tin of spam, or sausage or equivalent meat of your
  choice
- some grated cheese
- salt/pepper/garlic powder to taste

Empty the entire can of vegetable soup into a large bowl. Chop up
the meat into small chunks, as one might when preparing croutons,
for example (actual croutons are obviously a no-go here), and add to
the soup. Stir, then cover and microwave on High for 2 minutes.

After 2 minutes, add grated cheese to the dish and stir into the
soup, then cover again and microwave on High for another 2 minutes.
When done, stir in the seasonings and then serve. Simple as that!

* * *

The question of what to drink is a fairly simple one to answer, in my
estimation: water is fine. Though I have to admit that going straight
to water might be a bit of a leap for some, especially when the current
habits of many commonly revolve around sugary soft drinks and the
like. I should consider myself lucky that I was personally able to
break that particular habit separately back in 2010, long before I went
low carb with the rest of my diet.

I've never personally been into hot drinks like tea or coffee. In
fact, the only hot drink I consume regularly is a cup of water with a
teaspoon of chicken stock mixed in, then microwaved until hot; think
a quick and easy broth. And even then, that's generally only in the
winter. For me, cold drinks are my overall preference.

If I'm feeling like something more than just plain water, there are
various sweeteners that can be added to the water to give a little
flavour without going overboard; be it berry, blackcurrant, lemon or

lime. Any sweeteners based on a combination of stevia and/or erythritol are considered amongst the best, for their lack of insulin response.[6]

And for the really hot days, I can always make my own ice cubes or even entire blocks, by freezing that same flavoured water in a suitably shaped ice tray.

Snacks are something that I've pretty much phased out of my diet almost completely these days, but I certainly remember feeling the need for them during the earlier stages of my journey. When travelling I'll still sometimes pack a little something away with me, especially if I don't know when I'll next be able to find a spot for a suitable meal.

Snack options that I've used these last few years include hard-boiled eggs, pork rinds, macadamia nuts, salami, cherry tomatoes or frozen berries, the latter another nice cool option during the summer. And all of the above go really well with cheese, too.

Whether or not low-carb energy bars might count as a snack depends perhaps more on their size than anything else. For the little ones that are no more than two or three bites each, then sure. But occasionally I might have a larger one if I'm really out of options and I'm really hungry. They tend to hit the spot for a good while, but just like regular high-carb energy bars, they're not exactly whole, unprocessed foods, so I'll only have them occasionally.

When it comes to dining out, there are a number of options that I can enjoy. Most buffet restaurants are great, since I can just pick and choose the meat and veges that I know will suit. For something Asian I can have chop suey, or if I order a kebab it will simply be minus the wrap or the rice, leaving me with a simple plate of shredded meat and veges. No worries.

I'll also admit to a little fast food here and there, though I still have to be careful about it. The usual fries and drink combos I don't ever go near, of course, but there are other options. Many burger outlets will offer the choice of a lettuce wrap around their burgers in place of the usual bun. Others offer salad bowl options, with which

I'll usually ask for extra meat and cheese. And I'll even indulge in a bit of fried chicken now and then.

These things certainly aren't a focus of what I eat, though. Fast food is still just a once-a-week thing, as it always was for me while growing up. Why would that suddenly be an issue for me now? If anything, being able to still enjoy things like fried chicken now and then perhaps speaks to the efficacy of the rest of my diet, that I was still able to achieve what I've achieved, if not *because* of my eating some of these other things, but rather *in spite* of them.

Some can aim for perfection as much as they like, obsessing over food logs, apps to monitor macros and so on, but I've always kept things super simple in this regard. Again, my basic rules were just to eat to satiety, and keep the carbs to no more than 5g per 100g according to the label, and for me that was still enough.

And it's worth remembering the importance of personal sustainability for the plan as a whole, too. Whatever I can manage today, I have to be able to maintain tomorrow. Occasional treats such as these go a long way towards helping ensure that sustainability for me, while still staying near enough to the larger plan. That bigger picture is what really matters to me, and as long as that's still looking rosy, then I'm comfortable enough with my overall choices.

I don't have to get it completely right *all* of the time. I just have to get it right enough *most* of the time to still make a tangible difference, by whatever measure(s) I'm tracking over that time.

Or, put more simply: progress over perfection.

10 THE ISSUE, PART 1

I wonder where you got that idea from? I mean, the idea that it's feeble to change your mind once it's made up. That's a wrong idea, you know. Make up your mind about things, by all means — but if something happens to show that you are wrong, then it is feeble not to change your mind, Elizabeth. Only the strongest people have the pluck to change their minds, and say so, if they see they have been wrong in their ideas.
—*Enid Blyton,* The Naughtiest Girl in the School, *1940*[1]

FOR A GOOD WHILE during my active weight loss period around the middle of 2016, variations of the same single question would constantly come to mind, over and over and over: how is this low-carb thing not more widely known, not more widely understood, not more widely accepted than it currently is?

It was a question that I didn't dare to dwell upon for too long at any given time, for fear that I probably wouldn't like the answer. And at that point in my journey, I was determined to keep the mindset positive, to stick to looking after myself and sorting myself out, before considering the bigger picture.

And now, with enough time having passed for me to have finally had some opportunity to consider that bigger picture, I've come to suspect that my earlier fears are probably more justified than not.

In my experience, people have always been keen to learn how I lost the weight. Everybody wants to know the secret ... until I actually tell them. But it's only after the secret is revealed when things really start to get interesting, as individual reactions can differ wildly from person to person.

Some maintain their support regardless, as gamers typically would. They don't question the approach. All they care about are the results. All they care about is that it worked.

Others are enlightened by the revelation, admitting that they themselves might already have been curious about the approach, but were concerned at the mixed messages around its safety and efficacy, and are reassured with the knowledge that someone they personally know has actually made it work for them.

Some express a hint of disappointment, thinking aloud that they could never do the same thing themselves, out of what is sometimes termed online these days as FOMO: the Fear Of Missing Out. 'Oh, I couldn't bear to go without my bread', or 'but I love pasta'. Well, I ~~love~~ loved bread and pasta too, but it turns out that they don't love me.

Then there are those for whom the news represents a challenge to their very belief system as to what actually constitutes healthy eating. To them it's as if I 'lost weight wrong', that I 'got healthy wrong', or that, despite my results, 'my diet is still dangerous and will kill me', perhaps forgetting that at one point I pretty much had one foot in the grave already anyway.

Such a broad spectrum of viewpoints also appears to extend well beyond the level of the general public, deep into academia itself. This I came to understand for myself for the first time when I attended my first ever health conference in 2017. Throughout the day I spoke individually with four different speakers during the breaks, polling each of them for their views on nutrition.

One speaker was quick to invoke the words of author Michael Pollan. 'Eat food, not too much, mostly plants,' he told me. I offered a counterproposal, borrowing from the general paleo principle of eating real food, defining real food as anything that one would recognise as having recently been alive? He readily agreed with that, but he was dismissive of low-carb scientists, suggesting that at least one of them was motivated more by selling books than by the actual science itself.

I asked a second speaker about the sort of diet that she would choose to prescribe to overweight people, and the answer was traditional low-calorie fare, in general accordance with the guidelines. When I asked what her response would be to someone who had lost weight eating low carb instead, she frowned and replied that she'd want to know what their blood work looked like. So I rattled off my own blood pressure, HbA1c, triglyceride and HDL numbers. 'Oh ... well, I guess that sounds all right then,' she conceded begrudgingly.

A third speaker had discussed the mental health consequences of living with obesity. I found myself nodding my way through most of her presentation, and just had to tell her afterwards how much I could relate to many of the points that she'd made. Her answer to my question of preferred weight loss methods was interesting: 'You know, it's actually something I've known for a while that whenever I want to lose weight, I can just cut back on the carbs.' It was no big deal to her.

The fourth speaker I chatted with had made a point in his presentation about the motivational value of individual success stories. So I offered him mine: 50 kilos in 15 months on low carb, at which he seemed impressed.

The conversation continued, as I raised my frustration at how I had first heard about low carb years ago, but was scared away by experts of the time who had instead insisted that all I needed to do was just eat less and move more. He was nodding ever more vigorously as I spoke. 'Yeah. I almost feel like I want to apologise on behalf of my profession for having gotten things wrong for so long.'

Four different speakers, same conference; four different views, ranging from quietly cynical through to openly supportive.

The fact that they were all so different illustrated to me that, if nothing else, opinion plays a major hand in the formation of individual views, even in the minds of many of those whom the rest of us call experts.

I can't help but be fascinated at the ways in which these differences play out in the public arena. Thanks to the internet, we all have access to the same base of scientific literature; we just have to know where to look. And yet, different people will still inform themselves very differently, perhaps succumbing to their own confirmation bias, their desire to have their existing views reinforced, rather than challenged.

Of course, healthy debate on any subject is a good thing. But how healthy is the state of the debate over our nutrition? Perhaps the answer to that question is reflected in the extent to which we see our experts of today evolving their views over time. Which is to say, not greatly, which in turn suggests to me that the answer to the previous question is: not great. If anything, the landscape appears to have become more partisan, more divided than it has ever been.

Not only do many of these experts present conflicting positions to the public, but some will openly contest their positions with each other in battles for academic supremacy. And unfortunately, sometimes these interactions go beyond the boundaries of merely shooting the message, to shooting the messenger also.

Following the appointment of Prof Grant Schofield to a role with the Ministry of Education as Chief Education Health and Nutrition Advisor in April 2017,[2] one dietitian filed an Official Information Act request questioning the appointment process, out of concern for her perceived risk of 'greater confusion for the public and poorer health outcomes due to a lack of coordinated effort on childhood obesity,' given Schofield's research interests in what she described as 'areas of nutrition controversy.'[3]

More serious action has been taken for less. In 2015 dietitian Dr Caryn Zinn came under investigation by New Zealand's Dietitians Association, following a report against her by the Dietitians Association of Australia (DAA) concerning comments that Zinn made about low-carb diets on her own Facebook page. The Board's

Professional Conduct Committee considered the DAA's complaint and subsequently cleared Zinn of any wrongdoing.[4]

Targeted attacks by the nutrition establishment upon low-carb-friendly health professionals have occurred not just in New Zealand but around the world, from the case of Sweden's Dr Annika Dahlqvist in 2008,[5] to Australia's Jennifer Elliott in 2014,[6] to Canada's Dr Èvelyne Bourdua-Roy in 2017.[7]

In another Australian case, Dr Gary Fettke was anonymously reported to the Australian Health Practitioner Registration Agency (AHPRA) in July 2014, and then sanctioned by them in 2016. As an orthopaedic surgeon, Fettke is qualified to amputate diabetic limbs, but here he was effectively banned from providing simple nutrition information to his patients that may very well have served to save their limbs from amputation in the first place.[8]

This gag order persisted until September 2018, when AHPRA finally dropped all of its earlier charges against Fettke, issuing a written apology 'for the errors that were made when dealing with this notification', citing 'no evidence of any actual harm ... nor does the Board discern any particular risk to public health and safety moving forward.'[9]

Perhaps the best-known example comes from South Africa. In February 2014, researcher and author Prof Tim Noakes replied to a tweet asking if low carb was okay for breastfeeding mums, out of concern for 'all the dairy + cauliflower = wind for babies?' Noakes responded: 'Baby doesn't eat the dairy and cauliflower. Just very healthy high fat breast milk. Key is to wean baby onto LCHF.'[10]

For this single tweet, Noakes was reported to the Health Professions Council of South Africa (HPCSA) by the then-president of the Association for Dietetics in South Africa. In response, the HPCSA charged Noakes with 'unprofessional conduct for giving unconventional advice on a social network', in what became known locally as the 'Nutrition Trial of the 21st Century'.[11]

Across three different hearings held during 2015 and 2016, Noakes and his team presented many hours of testimony, covering a large body of scientific evidence supporting the safety and efficacy of an LCHF diet. Much of his case is freely available for viewing online.[12]

Noakes was found not guilty in April 2017;[13] in response, the HPCSA filed an appeal which was held in February 2018.[14] The committee's ruling — originally due before the end of March — was finally quietly announced late one Friday afternoon in June 2018, in which the charges were again dismissed by the committee and Noakes finally cleared of any wrongdoing.[15] The entire saga has since become the subject of his 2019 book *Real Food on Trial* with journalist Marika Sboros.[16]

The sum of these examples reflects a pretty serious situation, no doubt about it. From the outside looking in, it would be easy for most of us to simply view all of these different cases as the establishment heroically standing up for itself, defending the careful wisdom of the status quo against those who would challenge their prudent authority with delusions of half-baked quackery. Once upon a time I might even have believed that myself.

Except for this particular outsider, that status quo simply didn't work. It never did. If anything, that status quo may in fact have helped contribute to my chronic health issues in the first place. And in the end, it was the information provided by several of these very identities and others like them — effectively branded as renegades by many of their contemporaries — that finally led me to success.

So, what's a guy like me to think?

* * *

I solve problems for a living. Granted, they're not big, flashy glamorous problems by any stretch of the imagination. It's just software, it's just code. Typically, either someone will be requesting some new feature or functionality that doesn't already exist in the software, or they are raising some issue with what's already there.

Some problems are more complex than others. The simplest sorts of issues might merely involve corrections to grammar or punctuation. At the other end of the scale, some major feature requests can take months to turn around. Most jobs lie somewhere in between.

Generally when working on a given issue, there are a variety of ways in which I might be able to resolve it. Usually I'll come up with a few possible ideas as to the cause, and then work through that list starting with what I might consider to be the most likely cause, then the next most likely and so on, until I have found and isolated the actual cause. A similar process then follows with solution design options, starting with a design that is perhaps the simplest, most elegant, the least invasive to the existing code structure and working from there. Or sometimes it becomes worthwhile to consider a larger scale solution if time allows, for futureproofing purposes.

But sometimes I might get genuinely stuck on something. I might completely run out of ideas, or not have any at all to begin with. What happens then?

One Thursday morning in February 2018, I ran into a particular problem with a larger job that I'd been working on for a while. I'd written some code that was supposed to create a pair of new records in a database, one in each of two different tables. The tables in question had a direct 1:1 relationship, in that any record in one table should always have a corresponding record in the other table. The total number of records in each table should always be identical, and therefore the same sequence number should always be available to use when creating a new pair of records.

The problem facing me was that although the record in the first table was being created just fine, the second record refused to do the same; I was instead met with an error complaining that the sequence number in the second table was already in use. How could this be? All of the pre-existing records in both tables had consistently matching sequence numbers, so the sequence number that I had used to create a new record in one table should also have been available for the other.

After a good hour or so of fruitless debugging, I decided to apply one of my favourite pieces of advice that I picked up from the fictional Dr Gregory House of *House* fame years ago: 'When you run out of ideas that make sense, start looking at ideas that *don't* make sense,' the implication being that it's your own sense, your own understanding of things that's actually wrong.

It may only be one little thing within that understanding that may be off. At this point in my process I tend to ask myself: what other possibilities could come to light if I was wrong about this one thing, or this other thing? What else could emerge if any one of these things were different?

When I checked the tables themselves after running my code, I was expecting to find one new record in the first table only, since the error that I was getting seemed to relate to some issue with the second table. But to my surprise, both records had actually been created. It turned out that there was some undocumented behaviour in the system that automatically created a record in the second table, whenever a record in the first table was created. That's why I got the sequence number error, because it was already being used by the record that I didn't know it had already automatically created.

So I just needed to change my second instruction to update a record instead of creating it. From the code alone this would appear to make no sense, but I made a special note to properly document this area once it was all tidied up, so that this wouldn't confuse anybody else in the future. My understanding had been proven incorrect, but I learned from it and my understanding improved as a result.

In my line of work, I don't have the luxury of being able to wash my hands of anything that doesn't fit with my understanding of how things *should* work. My views have to evolve with the reality of the situation, not the other way around.

Overcoming one's own belief system can be incredibly difficult, especially if one is not used to challenging oneself in that way. Even with hard results staring back at me on the scales, it took me several more weeks to buy into the possibility that low carb might actually be working for me, because I'd had it drilled into me so deeply beforehand that it wouldn't.

Don't get me wrong, I can certainly understand how people can form their own ideas in the absence of quality evidence. The development of such hypotheses is a key step of the scientific method itself. The problem as I see it, is that once entrenched, some beliefs can take years to unravel again, sometimes long after evidence that dispels that belief has since come to light. Our innate desire for our beliefs to be true can sometimes blind us from our ability to recognise what actually is.

And the more authority held by people afflicted with such cognitive dissonance, the more contagious — and thus, the more dangerous — their view becomes. Would you believe a qualified mathematician if they told you that two plus two equals five, just because they were a qualified mathematician?

Such unwavering deference towards eminence over evidence, towards dogma over data, is nothing but a long-term exercise in futility. As more information comes to light about any given subject, we must all be prepared to update our own preconceived notions of how things actually work. What has been seen, cannot be unseen. And surely what has been seen, always ought to be worthy of explanation, no matter how controversial that explanation may at first seem.

Traditionally, when everyday people such as you or I look to address some issue with our health, we might go to our doctor or other health professional for information or advice. Beyond their own education, these professionals might themselves be further guided or informed by current health policy, which in turn one might expect to have been developed or informed by current science.

But then, who informs that science? Who watches the watchers?

I think the answer to that question ought to be you and me. All of us. We, the people. And I wonder if perhaps there's a bit of a missing link in what I feel ought to resemble some circular flow of information. That missing link is where I think the power of the individual experience can really shine.

What is science, after all, if not the means through which we seek to understand the phenomena that we observe in ourselves, the world around us and in worlds beyond?

We are all observers of our own environment. We are all our own n=1 experiments, our own case studies for the real scientists out there to draw upon, to inspire them to design and conduct their larger-scale studies, the results of which can in turn be picked up, referenced and applied by policymakers.

So why doesn't that happen more often? Given the current state of our wider public health situation, one would think that stories such as mine and hundreds of others around the world would inspire some added degree of curiosity on the part of researchers to explain this sort of success.[17] So where is that curiosity, and why haven't we seen that curiosity take shape in the form of more long-term studies on low carb?

When I personally asked one nutrition scientist that very question in front of a live conference audience in 2019, following his presentation (during which he himself had been critical of low carb), he assured those of us in attendance that the curiosity was definitely there, but as to why that curiosity hadn't translated into more studies: 'I simply don't know,' he finally answered.

I don't know either, but if history is anything to go by, I can guess.

* * *

It may come as something of a surprise at this point to learn that, to some extent, I actually do still subscribe to the standard energy balance model of calories in, calories out. If there wasn't at least some truth to the idea at some level, then there would be no such thing as the likes of Weight Watchers or Jenny Craig.[18] Such results-dependent organisations do not exist with the intention of going out of business.

The implications of the model when interpreted at face value, however, can be problematic. With a minimum of thought, one is quickly drawn to the same tired old conclusion that we've all heard a million times before:

Eat less, move more.

The issue I have with this statement on its own is that it provides no inherent clue as to how either of these things could be achieved on a sustainable basis. Telling a fat person to just eat less and move more is like telling a beggar on the street to just spend less and save more. As technically correct as this advice may be, it's also practically useless on its own. Beyond the question of just what to do lies the question of how to do it.

For some people, cutting back a bit at mealtimes and/or upping their exercise may be as simple a solution as is required. And if you can sustain and enjoy that in the long term, then that's fantastic. Have at it. All the best to you.

For the rest of us though, it's not quite so simple. While the energy balance model alone can explain a great deal for some individuals, it doesn't necessarily always answer the question when comparing people to each other. How is it that two different people can eat the same types and quantities of food, exercise similarly, and one gains weight as a result but the other doesn't? Or conversely, how is it that two people can eat the same food and do the same exercise, and one *loses* weight but the other doesn't?

To my problem-solving brain and me, the logical answer to that question would be that there's another influencing factor at play here. But what else could there possibly be? How, as traditionalists love to ask, can one possibly violate the laws of thermodynamics?

The answer to that question would be that the laws of thermodynamics aren't being violated as some would have us believe. The application of those laws to human physiology is simply being misunderstood.

The traditional energy balance model of calories in, calories out, asserts that by eating less and moving more, the body is compelled to make up for the shortfall of intake by mobilising existing fat stores for energy, resulting in overall weight loss.

In terms of what is eaten, the focus of this model is exclusively on quantity. But the quality of what we eat must also be taken into consideration. Otherwise we could just assume that 100 calories worth of carrots would be processed by the body in exactly the same way as would be 100 calories worth of cake.

This model, on its own, is incomplete. It ignores the very real consequences of inattention to the quality of our diet through the varied hormonal responses that can result, depending on exactly what one chooses to eat, when they do eat. Chief among those hormones is insulin, and this is what I've come to understand about how it works.

Insulin serves a number of roles in the human body, but is primarily responsible for keeping the amount of glucose in our blood down to a safe level. This is a very important job, as too much glucose in the blood can do considerable harm to the body over time. Type 2 diabetes itself is literally the disease state of chronically elevated blood glucose, and brings with it all sorts of terrible consequences if left unchecked, as too many of us already know.[19]

Under normal circumstances, the presence of excess glucose in the blood stimulates production of insulin by the beta cells of the pancreas. That insulin response then drives glucose back out of the blood, to wherever else it can find a home.[20] In this way, our insulin response can almost be considered a kind of biological safety net for our blood sugar control. Without it, most of us would have a diabetic crisis after almost every meal.

So where does all that glucose go?

The body's first choice — as directed by insulin — is that it be consumed immediately for energy. Some amounts of it can also be stored in our muscles and liver as glycogen, but in the grand scheme of things, our capacity for glycogen storage isn't terribly great. Beyond that, any excess glucose that can't be immediately burned or stored in its existing form is then converted by the liver into another different form entirely, a form for which the human body is only too capable of storing in seemingly limitless amounts: fat.[21]

Now, consider the implications of this. If the body is being directed by insulin to preferentially burn glucose for energy, then that preference will also come at the expense of the body's otherwise inherent ability to also burn fat for the same purpose. Combine that notion with the final destination for excess glucose also being fat, and it becomes apparent that the flow-on effects of insulin can result in a disastrous double-whammy for anyone looking to lose weight: insulin separately encourages the accumulation of new fat, as well as reducing our ability to burn existing fat, both at the same time.[22]

With this in mind, the potential problem for some people trying to follow a purely calorie-based approach to weight loss becomes clearer. If the body's ability to mobilise its own fat stores is being suppressed by insulin, then the only way to feed the body with energy that it can still recognise is through what we are eating. But if we are eating less in the presence of insulin, then suddenly a shortfall exists with only two other possible ways for the body to attempt to compensate: either by slowing down our internal base metabolic rate, leaving us tired and listless; or by telling us to eat more, through the signals of hunger; or both.[23]

So there's actually no violating of any laws of thermodynamics going on here at all. The body is always doing its level best to maintain energy homeostasis through the avenues that it has available. The problem is just that sometimes the avenue that matters to many of us the most — the fat stores that we all carry — isn't actually always available. If there's enough insulin going around, then it's as if our fat stores aren't even there at all.

This, I now believe, is what was happening to me when I was younger. I was prescribed a standard low-fat, low-calorie diet in keeping with the food pyramid of the day, and encouraged — sometimes forced — to move more, yet all that resulted was my getting more tired, and even more hungry.

I don't know that I would describe myself as ever having been addicted to food as such, since I do remember times now and then when I might not feel like eating. That would only happen though when I wasn't hungry, and those times were rare. My problem was more that for decades, I was almost constantly, uncontrollably hungry. In following the standard advice, I became, in effect, a slave to my hunger.

And then I think ahead to that bright sunny day at the cafeteria, when I instinctively got up for seconds, only to then realise that I didn't actually feel like seconds any more. And best of all, that's been the new standard for me ever since. One plate is still enough for me even now.

While nobody understood it at the time, it seems to me now that insulin may very well have been the potential missing link, the most likely answer to the question that I used to ask myself while walking home after school every day: why do I still get hungry when I'm already fat?

It still may not be fair, but at least now it all makes sense.

So let's work our way backwards here. To understand how to lower insulin levels in order to then be able to lose weight, we simply need to understand the process of how insulin is raised in the first place, so we can attempt to prevent or reverse that process. And since insulin production is stimulated predominantly in response to an excess of blood glucose, then examining the source of all that glucose would seem like a good place to start.

That starting point is really just the stuff that we put in our mouths. As many of us rightly suspect, it all comes down to what we eat, if perhaps not necessarily in the ways that we might currently understand.

Different types of foods contain different proportions of different types of macronutrients: fats, proteins and carbohydrates. As is already commonly known, fat is the most energy-dense of the three; a gram of fat contains nine calories worth of energy, while a gram of protein or carbs each contains four calories. This simple fact has long formed a key pillar in the foundational argument for eating low fat for as long as I can remember. Lose the calories by focusing on the fat, and weight loss must surely follow.[24] At least in theory.

But if calories were the sole concern in any diet, then that would imply that our bodies would respond in the same way to all of the various forms in which those calories can be delivered, regardless of what we may choose to eat. But we know that this cannot be true, otherwise there would be little point in classifying nutrients as fats, proteins or carbs in the first place. They'd all be the same.

Beyond energy density, the other vitally important difference that exists between macronutrients is the extent of the insulin response induced by consumption of foods dominated by each of those macronutrients. Fat hardly raises insulin at all. Protein can to some degree, depending on various circumstances. But by far the greatest insulin response comes from eating carbs.[25] Why? Because glucose itself is a carb, the single most common form of simple carbohydrate in existence.[26]

And it's not just in the sweet-tasting sugary carbs, either. The other digestible carbs, the grains full of 'complex' carbs that sat in the 'eat most' bottom section of the food pyramid for years, the starches, are mostly just long chains of glucose molecules strung together as well. Any of these carbs, when consumed, are quickly broken down into their constituent molecules, and that glucose soon accumulates in the blood as a consequence. And the more refined or processed the carb source is, the more quickly that breakdown process occurs, and so the faster and higher the blood glucose level spikes.

One of the simplest and clearest demonstrations of the effects of different foods on blood glucose levels comes courtesy of GP Dr David Unwin, whose infographics provide examples of various common foods and the impact that they have on blood glucose, by way of a translation into equivalent teaspoons of sugar.[27] The glycaemic response to a number of foods traditionally considered healthy — potatoes, bananas, bread, rice and cereals, for example — may be higher than you think.

So how much glucose is too much? Surprisingly little. The average adult human body contains approximately 5 litres of blood. At typical blood glucose levels of 4.5 mmol/L, this amounts to a total of just 4 grams of glucose across the entire bloodstream, the equivalent of roughly a single teaspoon of sugar.[28] And it doesn't take much more than that before the body responds with insulin to move that extra glucose on again.

Repeated glucose spikes will also do further damage over time. As the body becomes accustomed — or 'resistant' — to the insulin response that follows, more and more insulin becomes necessary in order to achieve the same degree of glucose clearance from the bloodstream. That glucose is continually locked away as extra fat, hunger and fatigue grows as the fat becomes harder and harder to unlock due to ever-increasing insulin levels, and once this state of hyperinsulinaemia becomes chronic, full-blown insulin resistance is born.[29]

In the long term, the consequences of insulin resistance can develop in different people in different ways.[30] If the pancreas can somehow manage to keep up with the increased insulin production requirements being forced upon it, then we get fatter, just as I did. If it can't, then our blood glucose spirals out of control and we get type 2 diabetes. If it can keep up for a while but is eventually overwhelmed later, we become overweight and then diabetic.[31] And if we treat our diabetes with exogenous insulin, then we are simply trading the extent of one problem for more of another: the high blood glucose is exchanged for yet more weight gain.[32]

None of these health outcomes are by any means desirable, as any of us who have experienced any of them first hand will tell you.

So it clearly stands to reason that when it comes to weight loss, rather than reducing our intake of fat as a concentrated source of energy, an alternative approach could be to reduce our intake of carbohydrate as a concentrated source of glucose, for its uniquely insulinogenic, appetite-stimulating properties. Insulin resistance itself can effectively be considered a manifestation of carbohydrate intolerance; a sad irony, when one realises that long-term carbohydrate consumption appears to be the primary driver of insulin resistance in the first place.

Or, as Harvard University endocrinologist Dr George Cahill once so elegantly concluded: 'Carbohydrate is driving insulin is driving fat.'[33]

* * *

Of course, it's one thing for a theory to stand to reason. But it's another thing entirely for it to be able to stand up to the scientific evidence.

Across our public health policy, much is made of the notion that all dietary guideline recommendations be 'evidence-based'. And to a large extent, they are. But it's also worth remembering that not all evidence is created equal. As Dr Jason Fung wrote in his 2016 book *The Obesity Code*, 'evidence-based medicine does not mean taking every piece of low-quality evidence at face value.'[34]

Evidence, in scientific terms, comes in several grades. Broadly speaking, study types can be divided into two groups: observational and interventional. Specific study designs within each grouping can also vary, and then there are meta-analyses — studies of studies — that attempt to paint an overall picture with regard to a particular issue.

Observational studies deal with the measuring of the extent of associations between one phenomenon and another, but generally aren't considered reliable enough to establish a causal relationship in any particular direction. The data can also be prone to various confounding factors, which typically then lead to retrospective adjustments to that data. While these studies can be used to generate hypotheses for stronger types of studies to examine more closely, the findings of observational studies themselves should not be overly relied upon by default.

In nutrition, observational studies are a dime a dozen. Most 'study of the day' headlines we might read or hear about in the news will tend to be observational, identifying weak associations at best, that may very well be refuted by another study soon after. Correlation is easily mistaken for causation in today's media. One day coffee is declared good for us, for example, the next it's not, and so on.

Meta-analyses of observational studies can lead to even muddier conclusions, with the pooling of studies that may individually indicate a positive or negative association to attempt to establish some kind of average outcome. But the various confounders — and resulting adjustments — soon add up as well. On this basis, coffee might turn out to be kinda-sorta good or bad for us ... maybe?

Interventional studies, on the other hand, consist of experiments in the form of trials. These trials are generally controlled for as many factors as possible, ideally through the randomisation of participants into two or more groups. Different interventions are then introduced to each of the study groups, with the aim being to establish the extent to which these different interventions may lead to different outcomes, with the potential for identifying a true cause-and-effect mechanism.

Nutrition trials in humans are notoriously difficult and expensive to conduct, which is why not so many of them exist relative to observational studies, and many that do don't always run for very long or have a smaller number of participants. Poor compliance is a major issue, particularly in randomised trials; unless a given participant happens to enjoy their designated dietary regimen, who wants to be told to eat a certain way for months at a time, with no guarantee of benefit at the end?

However, those larger, longer-term trials that do exist provide valuable information of a far higher standard than observational studies alone could ever hope to achieve. And meta-analyses of these trials are considered the pinnacle of scientific quality.

So with that all said, let's take a look at the trial-quality evidence examining the efficacy of low-carb diets for weight loss.

UK-registered charity organisation the Public Health Collaboration maintains a list of 67 randomised controlled trials (RCTs) on its website, comparing the results of low-carb diets against low-fat diets. Of the 33 trials listed that ran for a minimum of six months, twelve produced statistically significant results in favour of low-carb diets, while not one trial of any length favoured low-fat diets to any corresponding degree.[35]

One systematic review of 13 RCTs with a minimum duration of six months conducted from 2000 to 2007 comparing low-carb diets to low-fat, showed that after six months the weighted mean difference in weight loss favoured low carb over low fat by just over 4kg, although this difference decreased to just over 1kg in favour of low carb after 12 months.[36]

Another meta-analysis of 13 longer-term RCTs, this time with a minimum duration of 12 months, drew similar conclusions, with a weighted mean difference in weight loss of around 0.91kg more on low carb than on low fat.[37]

One of the larger studies included in both of the above reviews — the *A to Z Weight Loss Study* — was a 12-month trial comparing four different dietary patterns for weight loss, in which 311 overweight or obese women (BMI range = 27 to 40) were randomised to either an Atkins, Zone, Ornish or LEARN diet. The results showed that the Atkins arm presented with both the largest average weight loss (4.7kg vs 1.6kg, 2.2kg and 2.6kg, respectively) and the lowest attrition rate, suggesting a greater ease of compliance with low carb than with the other diets.[38]

In another two-year study — the *Dietary Intervention Randomized Controlled Trial* (DIRECT) — 322 moderately obese people, mostly men (average BMI = 31), were randomised to one of three diets: low-fat, Mediterranean, or low-carb. Of the 272 participants who completed the full two-year period, the mean weight losses were 3.3kg, 4.6kg and 5.5kg, respectively; a result made all the more impressive by the fact that participants on the low-carb arm were the only ones not calorie restricted, i.e. they were allowed to eat to satiety, whereas the others were not.[39]

One of the most remarkable studies comes from research organisation and medical service provider Virta Health, whose trial first began in 2017. 349 type 2 diabetics — the vast majority of whom were also obese and on medication for their diabetes — nominated for themselves either a continuous care intervention including a low-carb diet (average BMI = 40.4) or a usual care option (average BMI = 36.7). Primary outcomes to be assessed were HbA1c levels, weight and diabetes medication.

After one year, patients in the intervention arm lowered their average HbA1c from 7.6% to 6.3%, lost an average of 12% of their body weight, and reduced their diabetes medicine use, including insulin prescriptions.[40] After two years, intervention patients held their average HbA1c at 6.6%, average weight loss held at 10%, and medication usage further declined.[41] And even after three and a half years, the benefits continued.[42]

Some other studies suggest a lesser degree of certainty at first glance. In another two-year trial, 307 obese participants (average BMI

= 36.1) were randomised to either a low-carb diet or a low-fat diet, with both groups also receiving comprehensive behavioural treatment. Weight loss after two years was roughly 7kg in both groups, although lipid profiles showed a greater degree of improvement in the low-carb arm.[43]

The deck was possibly stacked a little against low carb in this instance though because, as with the DIRECT trial, participants in the low-carb arm were not calorie restricted, whereas those on low fat were. But in addition, the amount of carbs in the low-carb diet here was gradually increased after the first three months, which one can easily imagine might also have affected the results. Those sorts of details don't always make it to the headlines though, as the study's conclusion with regard to weight loss was simply that 'successful weight loss can be achieved with either a low fat or low carbohydrate diet when coupled with behavioural treatment.'

A similar sentiment was expressed following the results of another large meta-analysis of 48 RCTs, which compared a range of dietary patterns for weight loss. Low carb was found to have performed best after six months, though there was little difference between low carb and low fat after 12 months. 'This supports the practice of recommending any diet that a patient will adhere to in order to lose weight,' the study concluded.[44]

Proponents of the energy balance model above all else could interpret such statements as meaning that it therefore doesn't matter which dietary approach we try. But it's also worth remembering that study results generally reflect the study group(s) as a whole. Even if both a low-carb and a low-fat diet were considered equally effective at a population level, we are all still different as individuals. How might anyone predict which dietary approach could work out better for them at a personal level?

In a study performed as part of the *Comprehensive Assessment of Long-term Effects of Reducing Intake of Energy* (CALERIE) trial, 34 mildly overweight participants (average BMI = 27.5) were randomised to either a high-glycaemic load diet (60% of energy from carbs) or a low-glycaemic load diet (40% of energy from carbs) for six months.

The resulting data was then stratified according to the average level of insulin resistance, where it was found that while the insulin-sensitive participants actually lost slightly more weight on low fat than on low carb, those in the insulin-resistant bracket lost considerably more weight on low carb than on low fat.[45]

This particular finding really serves to highlight the importance of insulin and its effects on our individual capacity to metabolise energy from food in different forms, and ought to have us all wondering what our own levels of insulin might be.

Here in New Zealand, insulin unfortunately tends not to be something that is directly measured as a matter of routine, or at least is not included in typical blood work by default. From my own experience, it has to be requested specifically. However, in the absence of a direct measure, there are other easier-to-measure markers that can also give us a reasonable clue.

One study of various lipid markers and marker combinations as possible proxy indicators of insulin resistance showed that of the measures taken as part of a standard blood lipid panel, a high triglyceride (TG)-to-HDL cholesterol ratio was associated more strongly both with insulin resistance and with adverse cardiovascular outcomes than other markers, including the notorious LDL cholesterol.[46]

This suggests, in other words, that the higher one's TG:HDL ratio, the more insulin resistant one is likely to be, and thus, the more effective a low-carb diet may be for weight loss for that individual, than a low-fat diet.

And what's more, many of those lipid markers themselves also show substantial improvement on a low-carb diet. Another trial compared a wide range of markers for 40 participants (BMI > 25) randomised to either a low-carb or a low-fat diet for 12 weeks. Not only did participants in the low-carb arm lose more weight, but they also achieved superior outcomes in several markers including glucose, insulin, insulin resistance, triglycerides and HDL cholesterol, as well as for a range of other markers of inflammation.[47]

So it really does seem to me on the basis of all of this solid, high-quality evidence, that those of us with conditions resulting from an underlying state of insulin resistance, such as obesity or type 2 diabetes, may very well find that a low-carb diet could be at least as viable a dietary option as a traditional low-fat, low-calorie approach, if not more so.

Why then, after all that, do New Zealand's dietary guidelines not just fail to endorse a low-carb diet as a valid option, but actually explicitly advise against it altogether? According to a supplementary Ministry of Health document discussing a variety of topical issues around nutrition, 'there is no evidence of the long-term benefits or safety of such diets. Based on all the current evidence, the Ministry of Health does not recommend low carb, high fat diets for weight loss.'[48]

Something just doesn't add up.

11 THE ISSUE, PART 2

I am certainly not an advocate for frequent and untried changes in laws and constitutions, ... [but] laws and institutions must go hand in hand with the progress of the human mind. As that becomes more developed, more enlightened, as new discoveries are made, new truths disclosed, and manners and opinions change with the change of circumstances, institutions must advance also, and keep pace with the times.
—*Thomas Jefferson,* Letter to Samuel Kercheval, *1816*[1]

IF A PICTURE PAINTS A THOUSAND WORDS, then no doubt it says a lot that of all the images I can recall from my adolescence, few are so vividly, permanently seared into my brain as is the image of New Zealand's healthy food pyramid.[2]

Even now when I close my eyes, I can see it all, clear as day. The three layers of the pyramid, each shape outlined in black, all upon a stark white background. The food groups themselves, photographed onto the shape surfaces, with captions written on the outside, complete with accompanying orders, all barked in caps: 'EAT MOST: FRUITS, VEGETABLES. BREADS, CEREALS.' The Heart Foundation's *Eat to Beat* logo in the corner.

Perhaps the only thought that stands out in my mind even more clearly from that time than the pyramid itself, is the contrast of that pyramid and all of the advice that it contained, with the complete and total utter failure of that advice as an effective approach for controlling my weight.

For many years, I had always been of the view that I was to blame for my own predicament, that my failure to be able to do what seemed to come so easily — so naturally — to everybody else, lay with me and me alone. If I'm fat, then it's my fault.

And yet, when I was finally able to lose the weight, the realisation that it happened not because I kept trying to follow the standard advice, but only once I consciously chose to ignore that standard advice, has led me to become something of a sceptic of that advice. As a consumer, I feel that I ought to have confidence in the accuracy and integrity of such information. But as of late, I can't help but feel that that confidence has been seriously shaken.

And so finally in recent years, I began to explore the reason for this disconnect. How did this advice represented by various diagrams over the years, from pyramids to plates to star ratings to traffic lights, come to prevail in the first place, to take on its aura of established fact? What justification is there, in scientific terms, for the messages we continue to hear today about what constitutes a healthy diet?

Here in New Zealand, our dietary guidelines are administered by the Government's Ministry of Health, and are now called the *Eating and Activity Guidelines* (EAGs),[3] a reflection of the incorporation of recommendations around physical activity into what was previously a more diet-focused document. This in itself is a clue as to the overall thinking behind the guidelines. The classic energy balance model is in full display here; by this logic, it's okay if we eat too much, as long as we just exercise those surplus calories away afterwards.

My search for understanding began with an examination of the 2015 edition of those guidelines themselves.[4] And to be fair, there were a number of good points in there that were worth getting behind. The language placed a good deal of emphasis on whole, unprocessed foods over refined, processed foods. And sugar, as it always has, continued to be highlighted as an ongoing concern. So far, so good.

Some messages appeared to have evolved over the years since I was young, also. Where once the word on grains was universally positive, there was now some deserved recognition of the dangers of refined grains. Whole grains though, continued to be painted in a favourable light, a position perhaps more likely held on the basis of their reduced glycaemic impact relative to refined grains,[5] than on more absolute terms.

The best available evidence on whole grains for weight loss, however, is less encouraging. A meta-analysis of 21 different RCTs investigating the effects of whole-grain products or diets high in whole-grain foods, compared with a control diet, found no significant effect of whole-grain consumption on body weight, BMI, waist circumference or fat mass. Their findings 'did not support current recommendations of whole-grain intake in attempts to control obesity measures.'[6]

A further systematic review assessing the results of nine different RCTs comparing whole-grain consumption versus lower whole-grain or refined grain control groups, also found there to be 'insufficient evidence from those RCTs of an effect of whole grain diets on cardiovascular outcomes or on major CVD risk factors such as blood lipids and blood pressure.'[7]

And then there's the subject of fat. For so long, we'd been encouraged to eat low fat wherever possible. That message now, though, had finally begun to change, if not yet completely for the better. Rather than demonising fat as a whole, the emphasis now lay more specifically upon limiting our intake of saturated fat.

The rationale for doing so, however, remains elusive and, as it turns out, always has. In a systematic review and meta-analysis of six RCTs examining the relationship between dietary fat, serum cholesterol and the development of coronary heart disease (CHD), no differences in all-cause mortality were found, and no significant differences in CHD mortality were found.[8]

These six trials were all carried out prior to 1983, the year before the United Kingdom's dietary guidelines were first introduced, and so they represented the best available evidence on the subject at that time, on the basis of which a message of safety for saturated fat could have been delivered to the public. Yet, just like in the US a few years earlier, millions of UK citizens were instructed to limit their saturated fat intake instead.[9]

But that was then. What do we know about saturated fat now? Another similar systematic review and meta-analysis of 10 dietary trials, this time representing all of the best-quality evidence available as of 2016, again found no significant difference in all-cause mortality or CHD mortality, resulting from the dietary fat interventions. 'RCT evidence currently available does not support the current dietary fat guidelines,' the study concluded.[10]

Another important point worth noting is that, in both of these reviews, it was generally found that saturated fat did indeed have the effect of raising blood cholesterol levels (both HDL and LDL), but again, that increase in cholesterol had no significant bearing on mortality rates whatsoever.

Correspondingly, a further meta-analysis of four well-controlled RCTs examining the effects of replacing saturated fat in the diet with (mostly omega-6) polyunsaturated fat also found that, while those on the polyunsaturated fat diet did see a reduction in blood cholesterol levels as might be expected, there were still no such reductions to rates of CHD events, CHD mortality or total mortality. These findings were also said to 'have implications for current dietary recommendations.'[11]

Indeed. If saturated fat really was responsible for clogging our arteries with cholesterol and choking our hearts as a consequence, as had been so boldly proclaimed by experts back in the day,[12] then such outcomes would surely have been reflected in the results of these trials. But they weren't.

And yet in spite of this, we continue to be exhorted to consume low-fat dairy, to trim the fat from our meat and, increasingly, the meat from our diet altogether. The perceived risk specifically around red meat stems from sources such as the World Cancer Research

Fund (WCRF), whose report on diet and cancer prevention — most recently updated in 2018 — concluded that 'consumption of red meat is probably a cause of colorectal cancer,'[13] even though this statement was made on the basis of findings from observational studies only.[14]

The following year, however, a systematic review of randomised trials assessing the effect of red meat intake on cardiometabolic and cancer outcomes found no such relationship as suggested by the WCRF. 'Our results from the evaluation of randomised trials do not support the recommendations in the United Kingdom, United States, or World Cancer Research Fund guidelines on red meat intake,' going some way towards highlighting 'the uncertainty regarding causal relationships between red meat consumption and major cardiometabolic and cancer outcomes.'[15]

But the general narrative against meat continues to hold sway, all the same. Even the word 'meat' itself is becoming harder to find in our guidelines, as they now begin openly trending towards 'including more plant (such as legumes, nuts and seeds) and seafood-based protein foods in the diet.'[16]

It's worth making the technical point here that protein, like fat, is not actually a food: protein is a macronutrient. We don't eat nutrients, we eat foods containing nutrients. If we are to be guided on how we ought to eat, should it not be based either on conventional food groups or on nutrient distribution, but not both at once? These are separate measures, and so to mix the two can only confuse the picture further.

It would appear then that there are multiple barriers to the validation of low-carb diets within our guidelines. Not only is the concept as a whole discussed and disregarded on the basis of a purported lack of evidence that does in fact exist after all, but several individual components of a typical low-carb approach are also opposed, again in the face of quality evidence that strongly suggests the contrary.

All of which begs the obvious question: from where does the Ministry of Health gather its evidence, if not from a range of high-quality trials from across the scientific literature?

* * *

The EAGs themselves were accompanied by several supporting documents, all of which were worth a closer look. Between them, they described changes to the guidelines from previous incarnations, as well as addressing a range of other related questions.

One supporting document compared the statements of New Zealand's guidelines with those of other countries. 'The Guidelines Statements are based on the evidence that has been used to develop eating (dietary) and physical activity guidelines for a number of similar "developed" countries. The Eating Statements are similar to guidelines from Australia, the United States of America (2010 and information used to prepare the 2015 edition), and the Nordic countries.'[17]

Indeed, of the four international evidence sources cited for the eating statements in the EAGs, three were the equivalent dietary guideline documents for other parts of the world. Top of the list was the United States (2010), followed by the Nordic countries (2012) and Australia (2013).[18]

The problem with these particular sources, to me, is that they are effectively second-hand information. The guidelines of other parts of the world are not so much evidence in direct terms, as they are interpretations of the evidence, consensus statements, the carefully curated end products of their own respective review processes that each preceded them.

Imagine relying on a photocopy of a photocopy, or rounding off your numbers during each step of a complex series of calculations. With each successive iteration, more and more of the details get lost along the way, the further and further away from the source material we go. In this regard, New Zealand's guidelines largely serve as an interpretation of other interpretations of the evidence, somewhat removed from the actual evidence itself.

Ideally, the reference sources informing our guidelines would sit much closer to the underlying data. Otherwise, any possible flaws in any of these intermediary review processes could potentially be carried over and incorporated into our own guidelines.

Take for example the 2013 Australian guidelines. In a 2011 review of the evidence informing those guidelines, a 'dearth of evidence' was noted in terms of trials, 'and much of the scientific evidence is observational, especially from prospective cohort studies.' The solution? 'In some cases therefore, when assessing the overall evidence base used to establish grades for the evidence statements, a rating of excellent has been given when only [prospective cohort studies] are available.'[19]

In other words, while it was rightly acknowledged that much of the evidence that exists around nutrition is of lesser quality, that evidence was considered anyway, and even treated as if it were more reliable than it actually is. And then, by our Ministry's own review process, those results were reconsidered in turn.

For the Ministry to claim that its position on low-carb diets was made on the basis of 'all the current evidence', one might have expected a more thorough and direct process to have been carried out locally, a comprehensive New Zealand-based systematic review of the literature. Yet no such review appears to exist.

The reasons for this absence were suggested to relate to resourcing constraints. According to another supporting document, 'the Ministry's capacity for Guidelines development will never be as well-resourced as significantly larger and more populous countries such as Australia, the United States of America and the United Kingdom.' Consequently, 'the best option is for New Zealand to identify and consider the already completed international evidence or systematic reviews that underpin the dietary and physical activity guidelines of larger countries.'[20]

This might have seemed on the surface like a perfectly reasonable position to take, if the health outcomes of those other parts of the world were significantly better than ours. But Australia's obesity statistics are merely comparable to those of New Zealand.[21] The UK is only doing marginally better,[22] and the US is doing considerably worse.[23]

Of course, one could simply claim at this point in the discussion that it's not the advice itself that is wrong, it's that the people are just not following that advice. Many have made such claims over the years, often enough for me to have believed it for most of my life. But what does the data actually say?

The earliest New Zealand-based nutrition survey was the *National Diet Survey* conducted for the National Heart Foundation in 1977,[24] while the most recent was the *New Zealand Adult Nutrition Survey* conducted for the Ministry of Health in 2008/09.[25] While there are some variations and limitations in the data capture methods used across the different surveys over the years, the 1977 data set is the only New Zealand-based data set that exists from a time before the publication — and thus, any possible influence — of any government-level dietary guidelines anywhere in the world.

The 1977 findings were summarised in the survey's follow-up report in fairly blunt fashion. 'New Zealanders as a group eat too much. Too much of many things, but especially too much energy in relation to their expenditure, which of course must contribute in a major way to the genesis of obesity.'[26] The report's recommendations included 'increasing complex carbohydrate consumption as a proportion of total energy sources,' and 'reduction in total fat consumption,' variations of which have echoed on in successive editions of New Zealand's dietary guidelines ever since their introduction in 1991.[27]

So, how have we been doing over the years?

Comparing the data between the two surveys, New Zealanders do indeed appear to be eating less than before. The median daily energy consumption for males has reduced substantially, from approximately 13,551kJ (3237 calories) in 1977 to 10,380kJ (2479 calories) in 2008/09. For females, the numbers are approximately 8271kJ (1975 calories) and 7448kJ (1779 calories), respectively.

The changes in macronutrient percentages make for interesting reading, also. Carbohydrate consumption has increased markedly in males from 37.3% of total energy to 46%, and in females from 39% to 47.1%. Protein consumption has increased slightly in males from

14.6% to 16.4%, and in females from 14.9% to 16.5%. Fat consumption meanwhile has correspondingly decreased, in males from 41.5% to 33.7%, and in females from 43.9% to 33.8%. At this level, we've been doing exactly as we've been told.

Other statistics of note include those on sucrose (table sugar) consumption, the daily median of which has decreased slightly in males from 66.1g to 55g, but increased slightly in females from 38.2g to 42g. Fibre consumption has increased slightly in males from a daily median of 20.9g to 22.1g, and in females from 15.4g to 17.5g. And the much-maligned saturated fat has seen a considerable drop in consumption, from a daily median in males of 70.4g down to 36.5g, and in females from 46.4g down to 25.8g.

So on the whole, we've actually been doing remarkably well. Consumption of all three macronutrients now falls within the 2008/09 recommended ranges of 45–65% for carbs, 15–25% for protein and 20–35% for fat. We still have some work to do on the sugar front, but fibre is slowly climbing, and saturated fat is well down, though at 13.1% of total energy, still not quite within the 2008/09 recommended upper limit of 10%.

Still, as a population we've clearly been listening. Even if not every single box has quite been ticked, we have gotten much closer to the mark overall now than we were before. Given the positive overall direction, one might therefore have expected to see at least some improvement to our overall state of health over this period as a consequence.

Except of course, the precise opposite has occurred instead. In 1977 the median BMI for males in this country was approximately 25 and the female number was 23.8;[28] by 2008/09 the mean BMI figures for both males and females had reached 27.6.[29] The average New Zealand adult had become overweight, and another decade on, our mean BMI continues to climb, reaching 28.1 by 2020.[30]

While our total life expectancy rates have continued to trend higher over this period, increasing since 1977 in males by approximately 10 years and in females by almost 8 years,[31] our healthy life expectancy rates are showing signs of levelling off, increasing by less than one year in both males and females from 2009 to 2016.[32] Thus, our overall quality of life, in percentage terms, is actually now in decline.

In fairness, these are correlations only; there are a range of possibilities that could explain these trends. The general concept of the 'obesogenic environment' and its various components in physical, economic, political and socio-cultural terms has been discussed now for a number of years.[33] But when considered in terms of simple plausibility, what aspect of that environment could possibly be affecting the health of our bodies more directly, than the very substances that we take into our bodies, the food that we eat and drink?

On the strength of this data, one has to consider the likelihood that perhaps the problem might not be so much a case of the people having failed the guidelines, as it may in fact be a case of the guidelines having failed the people. And as this history suggests, if we simply continue to do what everybody else does, then can we not simply expect to continue to end up with what everybody else has?

* * *

The one international source of evidence for the 2015 EAGs that perhaps lay sufficiently closely to the scientific literature in my mind, consisted of a series of systematic reviews carried out by the United States Department of Agriculture (USDA), ahead of the publication of the 2015 edition of the *Dietary Guidelines for Americans* (DGAs).[34]

These reviews, published in March 2014, sought to identify relationships between dietary patterns and various health outcomes,[35] one of which focused on outcomes defined by measures of body weight or obesity.[36] This particular review to me seemed well worthy of closer examination; after all, there is no local equivalent. Perhaps it would be safe to rely on a source such as this, from a part of the world that's been doing this for longer than anyone else?

The conclusion statement from this review was that 'more favourable outcomes related to body weight or risk of obesity were observed when there was increased adherence to a diet that emphasised fruits, vegetables, and whole grains. Some studies also reported more favourable body weight status over time with regular intake of fish and legumes, moderate intake of dairy products (particularly low-fat dairy) and alcohol, and low intake of meat (including red and processed meat), sugar-sweetened foods and drinks, refined grains, saturated fat, cholesterol, and sodium.'[37]

This all made for fairly familiar reading. It really wasn't much different from the recommendations in New Zealand's own guidelines, and so certainly served to verify the influence of this review on our guidelines.

But for all the clear signs of consistency here, the question of accuracy remained. What of all of those quality trials demonstrating low carb as a viable option for weight loss? Where do they fit into the picture? To further understand what was going on, I had to dig a little deeper.

Chapter 4A of the USDA's systematic review document covered the subject of relationships between dietary patterns and body weight. A series of four related questions were posed, with separate literature searches conducted in response to each of them. The studies returned from these searches were each then subjected to a range of eligibility criteria to ensure that certain standards were being met across the board, prior to their actual evaluation in the review itself.[38]

In the end, a total of just 38 studies were found to have met all of the criteria for this review. Of those studies, only six were trials; the remaining 32 were all prospective cohort studies.[39]

Not one low carb trial made the cut. Instead, of the six trials that were included, most assessed variations of Mediterranean, DASH (Dietary Approach to Stop Hypertension) or low fat dietary patterns against standard control diets, with results generally finding in modest favour of each of the interventions.[40]

Considering that nutrition-related articles are currently being published at a rate of over a thousand per week,[41] the fact that so few studies were ultimately returned for this review demonstrates just how strict all of the combined eligibility criteria were, which, in general terms, is undoubtedly a good thing. But at the same time, the fact that the majority of studies that made it through were observational studies and not trials, suggested to me that perhaps some of those individual criteria were not without issue.

We already know of several low-carb trials, for example. Presumably there are further trials supporting other dietary approaches as well. Was the number of suitable trials out there really so small, that so much observational data also had to be included for such an influential systematic review as this? Were these 38 studies really the best that the academic world had to offer? The criteria themselves at this point warranted closer examination.

Many criteria were perfectly understandable at first glance. Subjects in each study must be human, for example; studies on animals were excluded. Articles must have been published in peer-reviewed journals, in English. In the case of trials, at least 30 subjects per study arm were required.[42]

Some criteria raised further questions. The inclusion of prospective cohort studies — despite their observational nature — was permitted, which certainly explained their heavy presence in the set of studies that were eventually considered.[43]

And curiously, only journal publication dates from January 1980 onwards were allowed.[44] The reason for this particular cut-off was not made clear, though it may be worth remembering that many of the aforementioned trials exonerating saturated fat were originally published prior to this date; 1980 was also the year that marked the publication of the first edition of the DGAs, at a point in time when the low-fat craze was reaching its peak. In any case, surely a well-conducted study is a well-conducted study, regardless of when it was published?

But two criteria in particular stood out from the rest. The first of these was that studies must include a description of the dietary pattern(s) consumed by subjects, seemingly in terms of the food groups themselves.[45]

This would be fine for patterns such as a Mediterranean diet, for example: think fruits, vegetables, whole grains, lean meat, nuts and seeds, olive oil, and so on. But patterns such as low-carb or ketogenic diets are typically characterised around a targeted distribution of macronutrient intakes instead: a given percentage of energy from carbohydrate, another percentage from fat, and so on. This criterion would therefore likely disqualify many studies of low-carb and ketogenic diets.

The second criterion of interest was that study subjects must be either healthy or at risk of chronic disease; studies on subjects who were hospitalised, diagnosed with disease, and/or receiving medical treatment were excluded.[46]

Consider what this would mean for studies of low-carb diets. Many are conducted on subjects diagnosed with type 2 diabetes, a clear failure of this criterion. The majority of low-carb trials are conducted on people who are overweight or obese, people who clearly have weight to lose. Remember the BMI numbers of the subjects from those earlier trials? Over 30, over 35, over 40? These people could hardly be described as being metabolically healthy, and so this would constitute another likely reason for the exclusion of such studies.

Were that the case though, that would also demonstrate an inconsistency with the application of this criterion, as some of the trials that did pass muster for this review, themselves featured subjects who were obese or hypertensive. Since obesity, hypertension and type 2 diabetes are all characteristics of advanced metabolic syndrome (more on metabolic syndrome in the next chapter), it would seem fairer to have considered studies on subjects afflicted with any of these conditions on an equal basis.

But perhaps the most controversial aspect of this entire review lay not with the eligibility criteria themselves, but with the literature searches that were carried out beforehand.

For this review, a range of scientific databases were searched during the early months of 2012, using a variety of search terms and key words, including specific terms for various dietary patterns. Those dietary patterns searched for were primarily Mediterranean,

DASH, vegan and vegetarian; with the occasional additional search for the likes of 'prudent', 'Western' and 'plant-based' diets.[47]

This immediately explained two key points. Firstly, it explained why the nature of the review's conclusions featured aspects of Mediterranean, DASH and plant-based dietary patterns so prominently.

But secondly, and even more importantly, this single aspect of the review alone explained the near total absence of references to any dietary patterns in the realm of low carbohydrate, ketogenic, paleolithic or carnivore. It appeared that the reason for a lack of endorsement of low-carb diets in this review, the primary reason behind the relative lack of low-carb science being assessed here at all ... was because no direct searches for any low-carb science were even conducted in the first place.

Thus, much of that science could not have been considered because, in the end, it was simply overlooked.

How this was allowed to happen remains a mystery. However, what should be obvious to anyone at this point is that no fair assessment of any dietary pattern — low carb or otherwise — could possibly be expected of any sort of review such as this, without there even having been any attempt to search for studies examining that dietary pattern.

The flow-on effects of such a critical oversight as this are considerably far-reaching, to say the least. This series of systematic reviews directly informed the 2015 DGAs themselves, which in turn guided the available food options for millions of Americans in schools, in the military, and in hospital care; and influenced the everyday food choices made by millions more.[48] And if New Zealand is also making use of these same reviews in formulating guidelines of our own, then who knows how many other parts of the world are also doing the same?

With issues such as these present in the EAGs' reference material, the Ministry of Health's consequential lack of endorsement of low-carb diets for weight loss is perhaps made more understandable. But it is not, in my view, made any less misleading.

'Is a low carb, high fat diet the best way to lose weight?' the Ministry asks.[49] Until the science is allowed to tell the whole story, who can really say?

* * *

In July 2020, the USDA's Dietary Guidelines Advisory Committee (DGAC) published its latest series of systematic reviews,[50] accompanied by a separate scientific report,[51] all ahead of the forthcoming 2020 edition of the DGAs.

Considering what had transpired six years earlier, this to me seemed like an ideal opportunity to learn what, if anything, may have since changed about the review processes, and ultimately the nature of what the 2020 DGAs — and possibly the next edition of New Zealand's EAGs — may have to say about diet and weight loss.

My own anticipation for the 2020 reviews was also shared by many others. Following the USDA's announcement that, for the first time ever, public comments could be submitted to the DGAC online,[52] the website was swamped with over 60,000 submissions by June 2020.[53] Corporate interests also weren't shy about defending and promoting their respective products; of those comments submitted by organisations, more than two thirds represented the food and beverage industries.[54]

The first of the reviews delivered by the Dietary Patterns Subcommittee sought to answer the following question: 'What is the relationship between dietary patterns consumed and growth, size, body composition, and risk of overweight and obesity?'[55]

The very first point to check this time around was of course the details of the literature search itself. There was certainly plenty of room for improvement here over 2014. Had things gotten any better this time around?

As it turned out, they most definitely had. Three scientific databases were searched during October and November 2019, but this time with a much wider variety of dietary patterns being covered. In addition to the patterns that were searched for last time such as

Mediterranean, DASH, vegan and vegetarian, the subcommittee's searches now also included the likes of low carb, high carb, ketogenic, paleolithic, low fat, high fat, high protein and low sodium.[56]

As would be expected, this expanded set of search terms returned a much wider range of studies for further evaluation. To this point, things were looking encouraging. But this newer, wider set of science would still need to survive the required eligibility criteria to come.

Those criteria themselves also showed some tentative signs of improvement in 2020. For example, the requirement that dietary patterns in each study be clearly defined, now included the option of macronutrient distribution as an alternative or addition to a description of food groups themselves. This was another important change for the better, no doubt, but not without the addition of another little wrinkle: this alternative definition was only allowed on the condition that measures of all three macronutrients were specified in the study.[57]

This would mean that if any otherwise perfectly relevant low-carb trials happened to specify the percentage of carbs being consumed by its subjects, but not the percentages of protein or fat, for example, then those trials would be excluded.

An explanation for this particular requirement is provided in the DGAC's scientific report. 'The Committee established these criteria in order to take a holistic approach towards answering the scientific questions, and thus, requiring the entire distribution of macronutrients within the diet, rather than a select macronutrient in isolation.'[58]

On reflection, this seemed to me like a somewhat short-sighted position to take. To exclude studies assessing a single macronutrient would be to pre-emptively discount the possibility that any single macronutrient may have something to do with issues of body weight or obesity. Saturated fat, for example — something even more specific — has already been considered in isolation for many years; why would the same not be permitted of any broader macronutrient now? For a review of this standing, the more comprehensive approach would surely have been to consider the effects of individual macronutrients, as well as any possible combination of those macronutrients?

The other issue from 2014 was around the health status of study participants, which had now also been adjusted. Those studies that enrolled some participants diagnosed with a disease or classified as obese were now allowed, but there was still no such luck for studies that exclusively enrolled such unhealthy participants.[59]

While this change did address the inconsistency identified in the previous review, the continued exclusion of studies assessing exclusively unhealthy subjects would appear sufficient to continue to disqualify several low-carb trials; again, remembering that many of them are conducted on subjects who are all generally overweight and/or diabetic. Why, after all, would anyone ever conduct a weight loss trial on healthy people who don't need to lose weight?

The DGAC's scientific report also offered a possible clue for this position. 'Of note, the Committee was not charged with evaluating the evidence for dietary patterns to treat disease,'[60] but again, with no further clarification as to what constitutes a disease in this context.

Of course, to exclude studies on subjects suffering from any sort of infectious disease makes perfect sense. But no insight was provided as to why studies on subjects with non-communicable diseases like obesity and type 2 diabetes were also excluded.

It would almost seem as if this criterion was actually intended to exclude weight loss trials by design. But then, seemingly as if just to make certain, the appearance of yet another addendum made things unequivocally clear: studies that exclusively enrolled participants classified as obese, with the aim of treating their obesity, were expressly excluded.[61]

Recall that the remit of this review was specifically to understand the relationship between what we eat and what we weigh. Yet, one of the criteria within that same review explicitly stated that studies designed to induce weight loss, despite such studies constituting perhaps the most topical aspect of the entire review... somehow didn't count.

If ever there was a place in the scientific literature where people like me might hope to find the ultimate answers to their weight problems, one might reasonably expect to find it here. And yet here, of all places, the subcommittee chose — through a different set of means this time, but to similar ends — to once again disregard the very same set of studies that could have proven most insightful to the countless millions of Americans who need help with their weight, most of all.

The justification for this? 'Studies that used hypocaloric or energy-restricted diets to induce weight loss in participants with overweight or obesity were excluded, as it is not possible to isolate whether outcomes were due to reduced energy intake, the proportion of macronutrients or dietary pattern consumed, and/or weight loss.'[62]

That may be true at face value. However, there are still a number of low-carb trials that demonstrated weight loss even when calorie intake was unrestricted. And even within the context of energy-restricted diets, it could still be that some macronutrient distributions may work more effectively than others in helping to lose weight, or even that some compounding effect from a combination of the two approaches might exist. But without said weight loss trials having been included here at all, ideas such as these could not have been explored.

And on top of all of that, study design inclusion criteria had also been further loosened, with retrospective cohort studies and nested case-control studies being added to the list of acceptable designs,[63] thereby further increasing the potential influence of weaker, observational data. But by this point in the investigation, issues such as these were largely academic. The real damage had already been done.

Against the odds, a handful of studies labelled as low carb did somehow manage to survive all of these criteria. But on closer inspection, it turned out that they were effectively low carb in name only. All but one of those studies included failed to consider carb consumption below even 35% of total energy; most assessed carb levels of closer to 40%.[64]

In absolute terms, these aren't low-carb numbers at all, certainly nowhere near the much lower proportions being tested in several of the low-carb trials that were excluded. But those numbers were deemed as such here, on the basis that current recommendations suggest a minimum of 45% of total energy intake from carbohydrate,[65] the same minimum as that which was specified in the 2008/09 New Zealand Adult Nutrition Survey. Anything below this accepted minimum was therefore defined in this review as being 'low carb'.

This 45% minimum value appears to originate from a 2005 report on dietary reference intakes published by the National Academy of Sciences, Engineering and Medicine (NASEM).[66] Here, the figure seemed to have been estimated not so much on the basis of any particular concern about low carb, but more as a consequence of the reported dangers of a high-fat diet: 'high fat diets are usually accompanied by increased intakes of saturated fatty acids, which can raise plasma LDL cholesterol concentrations and further increase risk for CHD.' This, along with more general concerns about increased total energy intake on a high-fat diet, led more directly to a recommended upper limit for fat consumption of 35%, which, in combination with protein recommendations, led to the 45% minimum for carbohydrate coming about almost by default.[67]

On the subject of carbohydrate consumption more specifically, the NASEM report did suggest a minimum of 130g per day in order to provide the brain 'with an adequate supply of glucose fuel without the requirement for additional glucose production from ingested protein or [fat].'[68] Elsewhere though, the report stated that in individuals fully fat-adapted, such as they would be on a low-carb diet, 'ketoacid oxidation can account for approximately 80 percent of the brain's energy requirements.'[69] Most tellingly, the report even noted that 'the lower limit of dietary carbohydrate compatible with life apparently is zero, provided that adequate amounts of protein and fat are consumed.'[70] Yet, this observation was not at all reflected in the report's recommendations.

The age of the NASEM report itself — now over a decade and a half old — also predates much of the evidence in support of low carb that has accumulated in the years since. One can only imagine what an updated edition of this report might have to suggest about minimum carbohydrate consumption today.

In the end, the conclusions resulting from the 2020 USDA review were similar to its predecessor, which again declared that 'dietary patterns emphasizing vegetables, fruits, and whole grains; seafood and legumes; moderate in dairy products (particularly low and non-fat dairy) and alcohol; lower in meats (including red and processed meats), and low in sugar-sweetened foods and beverages, and refined grains are associated with favorable outcomes related to body weight (including lower BMI, waist circumference, or percent body fat) or risk of obesity. Components of the dietary patterns associated with these favorable outcomes include higher intakes of unsaturated fats and lower intakes of saturated fats, cholesterol, and sodium.'[71]

One notable change this time around was the addition of a second conclusion statement, which applied specifically to dietary patterns characterised primarily by their macronutrient distribution, including low carb. 'Insufficient evidence is available to determine the relationship between macronutrient distributions with proportions of energy falling outside of the acceptable macronutrient distribution range for at least one macronutrient and growth, size, body composition, and risk of overweight/obesity, due to methodological limitations and inconsistent results.'[72]

These conclusions could really only be considered accurate under the methodological confines through which they were formulated. Of course to claim a lack of evidence of low carb for weight loss makes perfect sense, when one's review criteria all but ensures that much of that evidence is ruled ineligible along the way. While it could be argued that this was technically still a better result than 2014 on the grounds that the subcommittee did at least search for low-carb studies this time around, that would have been a pretty low bar to have surpassed under any reasonable circumstances.

In December 2020, the latest edition of the *Dietary Guidelines for Americans* was finally published, to apply during the 2020–2025 period.[73] On the back of the preceding round of reviews, flawed as their underlying processes were, with it came continued recommendations for consumption of fruits, vegetables and grains, low-fat dairy, 'protein foods' and oils; and to limit consumption of foods containing added (not total) sugar, saturated fat, salt and alcohol.[74]

That very same month, the Ministry of Health published the 2020 edition of New Zealand's *Eating and Activity Guidelines*.[75] And on the basis of largely the same evidence sources as the 2015 edition, they too continued to recommend a diet of fruits, vegetables and grains, low-fat dairy, and some amounts of legumes, nuts and seeds, seafood, eggs, poultry and lean red meat ('protein foods'), while still favouring unsaturated fat over saturated fat, and also advising against the likes of added (not total) sugar, salt and alcohol.[76]

The more things change, the more they stay the same.

12 THE FUTURE

In the end, dietitians who continue to label LCHF as "dangerous" will simply be ignored by the informed public. Same with medical doctors. The marketplace will ultimately drive change. If it doesn't work and something else does, then the public will choose only that which works.
—*Prof Tim Noakes, Twitter, 2017*[1]

SOMETIMES I LIKE to imagine where the human race might be, say hundreds or even thousands of years into the future. To our distant descendants we are nothing more than the sum of our memories and experiences that we have preserved for posterity, historical references to be studied, the classical tales of their time.

I wonder what those people would think of us, based on what they would learn from what we leave of ourselves behind. They would surely be able to learn at least as much about us as what we have learned about those who have come before. The notion that there was ever a point in time at which there was so much contention over the ideal balance of nutrients in our diets in the first place, may seem just as patently absurd to those who will follow us in our future, as the debate over tobacco from our more recent past, for example, seems to us now.

I imagine they might look back at our time with a sense of bewilderment, at the fact that we seem to have lost a certain sense of perspective with regard to how and what to eat; that we had somehow managed to unlearn over the course of the latter half of the 20th century what had once been considered a simple, instinctive, practical, common sense understanding of how to most effectively address the issue of obesity; an already-established norm, supported by literature that now dates back almost two hundred years.

Among the earliest written records describing the relationship between carbohydrates and obesity is a book by French lawyer and politician Jean Anthelme Brillat-Savarin called *The Physiology of Taste*, first published in 1825 and translated into English several times in the years since.[2] The book was largely a philosophical discussion around the culture of food and the social pleasures associated with its preparation and consumption, but also touched on the subjects of both weight gain and weight loss.

His initial observation of the topic of obesity in humans was based on his reflections of the same phenomenon as it occurred in other species. 'I elucidated a theory whose elements I had first elucidated outside of mankind,' he wrote, 'namely that the chief cause of corpulence is a diet with starchy and farinaceous elements; and in this way I satisfied myself that the same diet is always followed by the same effect.'[3]

From these observations, Brillat-Savarin settled in his mind upon two principal causes of obesity, the first he described as a 'natural constitution of the individual,' accepting that all of us are born with various predispositions. 'It is certain therefore that there are persons virtually doomed as it were to corpulence, persons whose digestive activities, all things being equal, create more fat than those of their fellows.'[4]

His second cause of obesity was 'the floury substances which man makes the prime ingredients of his daily nourishment,' reminding readers that 'all animals that live on farinaceous food grow fat willy-nilly; and man is no exception to this universal law.'[5]

In treating the condition, diet was declared to be the most

important of factors, more so than either quality sleep or regular exercise. 'An anti-obesic diet must be governed by the most common and active cause of obesity,' he wrote, and so therefore, 'it may be inferred, as an exact consequence, that a more or less strict abstinence from all floury or starchy food leads to a diminution of flesh.'[6]

Brillat-Savarin's ideas were similar to those put forward by French physician Jean-François Dancel, whose own book *Obesity, or Excessive Corpulence* was published in 1864 and translated into English by 1873.[7]

Like his predecessor, Dancel observed that the extent of certain predispositions varied between individuals. 'We meet with many who do all in their power to grow fat, and who still remain thin,' he wrote, 'because, no doubt, they possess some peculiarity of organisation which prevents the development of fat.'[8] He also noted the increased prevalence of a variety of other health issues occurring alongside obesity, including headaches, swelling in the legs, fatty liver and skin diseases.[9]

But the more direct cause of obesity was claimed to be found in the character of one's food. Dancel was sceptical of plant-based diets, because in his professional experience, '[these] very means which have been recommended to overcome [obesity], are exactly those best fitted to induce and maintain it.'[10] While acknowledging that 'man can simultaneously feed upon both vegetable and animal matter,' his preferred treatment option for obesity was that 'without affecting the general health, the patient must feed chiefly upon meat.'[11]

At about the same time that Dancel's work appeared in France, so too did the writing of retired English undertaker William Banting, whose booklet *Letter on Corpulence* was first published in 1863. Such was the popularity of his work with the general public to whom it was directly dedicated, that several subsequent editions were released throughout the 1860s and beyond.[12]

Banting's was a remarkable personal success story of how he had initially struggled in dealing with a slow but steady weight gain throughout his middle and later years. He was told to eat less — 'moderation and light food was generally prescribed' — which left him feeling sickly and weak. He was told to move more, so he took up a rowing habit for two hours a day, which left him feeling tired and hungry.[13]

Finally one desperate day, he 'found the right man' in physician Dr William Harvey, who advised him to abstain from bread, butter, milk, sugar, beer and potatoes; all of which Banting had been consuming freely to that point. These foods, Harvey told him, 'contain starch and saccharine matter, tending to create fat, and should be avoided altogether.' Banting's new daily plan instead featured several helpings of various meats, some vegetables with the exception of potato, small amounts of fruit and dry toast, and a few glasses of wine. Across the 13 months from August 1862 to September 1863 he lost 46 pounds, the first 35 at an average of one pound per week.[14]

Banting's only lasting concern with this diet was of reticence from the academic community, in spite of its demonstrated effectiveness. 'Oh!' he lamented, 'that the faculty would look deeper into and make themselves better acquainted with the crying evil of obesity — that dreadful tormenting parasite on health and comfort. Their fellow men might not descend into early premature graves ... and certainly would not, during their sojourn on earth, endure so much bodily and consequently mental infirmity.'[15]

The so-called Banting Cure became so widely known in subsequent years that it was later referenced by Polish-German physician Dr Wilheim Ebstein in his book *Corpulence and its Treatment*, first published in 1882 and translated from the original German into several other languages including English by 1884.[16]

Like Dancel before him, Ebstein noted the association of obesity with a range of other conditions, in this instance anaemia, gout and diabetes;[17] he also identified several possible risk factors for obesity including genetics, the specific life stages of puberty and menopause, a lack of exercise, lack of sunlight, increased alcohol consumption and overeating in general.[18]

Of the nature of food itself, Ebstein wrote that the formation of fat is 'promoted to a prominent degree by the carbohydrates.' While he accepted that a range of dietary options existed 'by which a stout person may be made lean in a relatively short time,' he also emphasised the importance of a 'permanent change of habits,' beyond just the quick-fix solutions. Ultimately, Ebstein also advocated for a diet requiring 'exclusion of the carbohydrates,' but freely allowing the consumption of fat as it naturally occurred 'in the flesh,' for its observed tendency to induce satiety.[19]

As the turn of the century approached, the low-carb concept was becoming more and more well established. In 1892 Canadian physician Sir William Osler published the first edition of what would become an internationally renowned medical textbook — *The Principles and Practice of Medicine* — for decades to come. By 1912 the book had reached its 8th edition, having generally undergone revisions on a triennial basis until the onset of the First World War.[20]

Osler recognised both the physical and mental distress that obesity was capable of creating, and observed that its cause 'is not always due to excessive intake of food; many stout persons are light eaters. On the other hand, there are cases in which the increase in weight is directly due to an excessive consumption of food.'[21]

Something else was clearly at play as well. 'Fat metabolism is as yet imperfectly understood; it is under the control of the internal secretions,' he wrote. 'We see the deposition of fat in connection with many processes with which the internal secretions are concerned,' citing puberty, castration, menopause, pregnancy and lactation, as examples of life stages or events during or after which weight tends to increase.[22]

Osler's treatment for obesity was through regulation of the diet, not allowing children to eat sweets, and for women 'particularly to reduce the starches and sugars.' The proposed dietary plan was largely meat-based, allowing some fruit and vegetables 'without sugar,' and only a very small amount of bread.[23]

The common themes that emerge from each of these historical accounts are evident. For almost a hundred years by this point, there was very little debate that carbohydrates — both sugar and starch — were consistently seen to be fattening, and that to lose weight therefore meant a reduction or elimination of those carbohydrate-containing foods from the diet.

The authors behind these accounts also accepted the limits of their own understanding of the issue, particularly when it came to influences driven by the inner workings of the human body. It was often recognised that some people were more naturally predisposed to weight gain than others, and this was generally explained through the hypothesised presence of some hidden internal biochemical mechanism, the specifics of which had, so far, eluded them all.

That mystery would finally be solved in 1921, with the co-discovery by Frederick Banting — himself a distant relative of William Banting[24] — and Charles Best, of the hormone insulin.[25]

Fast forward another hundred years or so, to a point where our current understanding of the effect of insulin on our weight is perhaps best summarised as what has been called the carbohydrate-insulin model of obesity, submitted in 2018 as an alternative to the conventional energy balance model by Harvard Medical School endocrinologist and researcher Dr David Ludwig.[26]

The carbohydrate-insulin model (CIM) proposes that changes in our diet over the last several decades have led to changes in our collective hormone response, which in turn has led to greater proportions of energy contained in the food that we eat, to be stored as fat. And if more is being stored, then less is being burned, leaving us tired and/or hungry, thus the end result being a decreased desire to exercise and/or an increased desire to eat.

The parallels between the CIM and the energy balance model are striking. Both describe a similar series of steps, except for one critical difference in that the direction of causality is reversed. Instead of getting fat because we eat too much, this model essentially argues that we eat too much because we're getting fat. Though it may seem a counterintuitive idea at first, the CIM would appear to align well with a range of experiences documented across history, as well as explaining the successes observed in more recent low-carb trials, particularly those trials in which calorie intake was unrestricted.

'Primary emphasis should be placed on the *quality* rather than *quantity* of calories consumed,' the article recommends. In this context, the CIM suggests the glycaemic load (GL) of food as an effective measure of its quality: the lower the GL, the better. The GL of food is determined by its carbohydrate content multiplied by its glycaemic index (GI), the latter being a measure of how quickly a given food increases one's blood glucose levels, and in turn, the extent of our insulin response.[27]

Under this model, some of us may be more or less tolerant of higher-GI foods than others, and some of us may be more or less tolerant of higher-carb foods than others. A degree of experimentation to establish one's own personal tolerance levels is still allowed for. But too much of foods that measure highly in either GI or in carbs are advised against, and too much of foods that measure highly in both will tend not to end well for most of us.

And what foods might those be? Generally speaking, those that predominate a processed food diet. Think bread, grains and pasta, breakfast cereals, cakes, biscuits, pies and pastries, desserts, sweets, alcoholic and non-alcoholic sugary drinks; foods that contribute a combined total of over 50% of total energy to the typical daily New Zealand diet,[28] essentially the same foods that have been understood to be bad for our waistlines for the better part of two centuries.

We have the knowledge. It turns out we've had it all along. Even if we didn't have all the details figured out at first, we knew well enough to go along with it at the time, because we could tell for ourselves, time and time and time again ... that it worked.

Now we just need to apply that knowledge once again.

* * *

It's a curious thing, given our prior affinity for low carb, that the low-fat approach to losing weight — as inspired by the conventional energy balance model — is so well known, and yet for so many of us, it seems so difficult to apply in practice. Even more so, that our collective faith in the concept has remained so watertight, despite our collective failure to actually make it work.

I can admit, there is a certain allure about its simplicity. And on its own merits, low fat most certainly can and does work for a number of people. We see that, even in studies where low carb is found to be more favourable for weight loss overall, some individuals within those studies do find low fat to be genuinely more effective for them. That is not in dispute here. What is in dispute is the idea that weight loss must be as simple as that for everybody, that this one solution magically fits us all like a single universal glove. If only such a beautiful hypothesis were to hold true. But such is 'the great tragedy of science,' as described by biologist Thomas Huxley in 1870, that being 'the slaying of a beautiful hypothesis by an ugly fact.'[29]

Of course, we now understand that the issue with the low-fat approach is that it tends to work best only in the absence of insulin resistance, with its innate power to otherwise thwart the sincerest of efforts on the part of many of us to improve our metabolic health. But that hasn't stopped some scientists from actively pursuing the idea over the years anyway, even if the results weren't always quite so strong as have sometimes been portrayed.

The roots of the modern low-fat diet movement can be found in the quest to understand the cause of heart disease, a condition whose steadily increasing prevalence during the mid-20th century was in turn commanding increasing attention from the scientific community at that time.

In 1953 physician and researcher Dr Ancel Keys published an article titled *Atherosclerosis: A Problem in Newer Public Health*, in which he presented a graph demonstrating what appeared to be a powerful association between fat consumption and rates of heart disease deaths in men across six different countries. The association also grew stronger with age.[30]

The connection between the two trends was considered to be blood cholesterol levels; if cholesterol was a factor in heart disease, and if dietary fat raised cholesterol levels, then a diet lower in fat might therefore be helpful in preventing heart disease. The idea that blood cholesterol was somehow linked to atherosclerosis was not a new one even then — molecular scientist Dr John Gofman had explored this already with his 1950 discovery of three separate classes of lipoproteins: HDL, LDL and VLDL[31] — but it was Keys who first connected the dots of dietary fat with heart disease via cholesterol and, in doing so, set in motion a whole new wave of scientific interest in this area.

Unfortunately for Keys and his diet-heart hypothesis, as it came to be known, the six countries' worth of data that he had presented was but a fraction of the 22 countries for which such data was available at the time. When the full data set was published by Drs Jacob Yerushalmy and Herman Hilleboe in 1957, it showed the association between fat consumption and heart disease mortality to be far weaker, no better than a similar weak association for animal protein. Not only that, but it also showed that both fat and animal protein were negatively associated with *non*-cardiac disease. When viewed from a total health perspective therefore, it effectively all came out a wash.[32]

At about the same time in 1957, another paper by Dr John Yudkin highlighted the dangers of attempting to present such observational data as being indicative of causation, with data from his native UK also demonstrating heart disease rates increasing not only with sugar consumption, but also with ownership of radios, televisions and motor vehicles.[33]

Rather than being humbled by the criticism of his work, however, Keys was instead galvanised by it. Later that same year he published another paper, this time refining his hypothesis to focus more specifically on saturated fat, for its observed tendency to raise blood cholesterol levels, while polyunsaturated fats were now seen to lower it. Thus in order to lower cholesterol, removing saturated fat 'has the greatest effect, and this effect may be enhanced by substitution of such oils as corn oil and cottonseed oil,' Keys wrote.[34]

His cause was also given further exposure by the plight of US president Dwight D. Eisenhower, who himself had suffered the first of a series of heart attacks beginning in 1955. The treatment incorporated a strict diet low in both fat and cholesterol, as prescribed by his attending cardiologist Dr Paul Dudley White, an open supporter of Keys' work.[35]

Aided by this whole new level of publicity that now reached directly into living rooms across the nation, Keys' ideas and influence continued to spread. By 1961 he had the ear of the American Heart Association (AHA), who issued a statement in February of that year recommending a diet that both reduced total fat, and replaced saturated fat with polyunsaturated fat 'as a possible means of preventing atherosclerosis and decreasing the risk of heart attacks and strokes,' for anyone who was overweight, had a family history of heart disease or who was suffering from heart disease themselves.[36]

Throughout the 1960s Keys continued to pursue his hypothesis with a relentless determination, his efforts finally culminating in 1970 with the publication of his best-known body of research, first as a special issue of the AHA's journal *Circulation*, then as its own monograph in April of that year, titled *Coronary Heart Disease in Seven Countries*.[37]

For this study, Keys selected seven countries around the world, across parts of which he established teams of local researchers in Finland, Greece, Italy, Japan, the Netherlands, the United States and the former Yugoslavia. A combined total of 12,770 men aged 40 through 59 years were physically examined and their diets surveyed, then were reassessed five years later.

The published findings were more or less in line with what Keys had proposed through his earlier work. 'The incidence rate of CHD tends to be directly related to the distributions of serum cholesterol values,' he noted, and since 'the average serum cholesterol values of the cohorts tended to be directly related to the average proportion of calories provided by saturated fats in the diet,' the results seemed to validate the diet-heart hypothesis, that saturated fat in the diet was an implicating factor in the prevalence of heart disease.[38]

If there was any apparent weakness to the Seven Countries study, it might have been its design as another observational study, as opposed to being a trial. This was reflected in the findings of a 1971 report by the US National Heart and Lung Institute (NHLI), which recommended a range of clinical trials be carried out in order to test this and other hypotheses.[39] Some researchers already had trials under way by then anyway, with every intention of confirming the diet-heart hypothesis, and in turn, the diet low in saturated fat that could be suggested as the logical solution. The results of several of those trials, however, would turn out to be somewhat less than convincing.

One such study was the Sydney Diet Heart Study, a trial involving 458 Australian men aged 30–59 years with pre-existing heart disease, but who had also already made some degree of lifestyle change following their respective diagnoses. The trial began in 1966 and randomised participants to either a diet containing 13.5% saturated fat and 8.9% polyunsaturated fat, or a diet of 9.8% saturated fat and 15.1% polyunsaturated fat.

After five years of follow-up, it was found that both groups had lost similar amounts of weight and both groups had lowered their cholesterol, although the cholesterol reduction was greater in the low-saturated-fat group. However, there were also more deaths in the low-saturated-fat group, quite the opposite of what might have been predicted at the time.[40]

In the resulting journal article eventually published in 1978, the study authors suggested that other surrounding lifestyle changes among participants such as reduced smoking, weight loss and increased physical activity, may have outweighed the potential benefits of reducing saturated fat in the diet. A later re-evaluation of the original data in 2013, however, was far more direct in its conclusion: that replacing saturated fat with polyunsaturated fat 'did not provide the intended benefits, but increased all-cause mortality, cardiovascular death, and death from coronary heart disease.'[41]

Another much larger trial — the Minnesota Coronary Survey — began in November 1968 and ran for four and a half years, involving over 9000 institutionalised men and women across six Minnesota state mental hospitals and one nursing home. Participants were randomised to either a typical control diet containing 18% saturated fat and 5% polyunsaturated fat, or a treatment diet of 9% saturated fat and 15% polyunsaturated fat which featured products such as egg substitutes, margarine and low-fat beef with added vegetable oil.

The study showed that while total cholesterol was reduced by an average of 14.5% on the treatment diet versus only 0.7% on the control, this again did not translate to any significant reduction in cardiovascular events or total deaths from the treatment diet; in fact, just like Sydney, there were more deaths among the treatment group by trial's end than there were among the controls.[42]

Incredibly, these findings were not published until 1989, a full 16 years after the study's original conclusion. When study director Dr Ivan Frantz was later asked for an explanation for the delay, he simply answered: 'We were just disappointed in the way it came out.'[43] Another reassessment of this study in 2016 explained Frantz's disappointment more fully, concluding that replacing saturated fat with polyunsaturated fat does indeed lower cholesterol, but this 'does not support the hypothesis that this translates to a lower risk of death from coronary heart disease or all causes.'[44]

Still, the search for proof continued. Beginning in December 1973, the Multiple Risk Factor Intervention Trial (MRFIT) randomised 12,866 high-risk men aged 35 to 57 years to either a special intervention dietary plan requiring a reduction in saturated fat down to 10% of calories (later revised down to 8%) and increasing polyunsaturated fat intake to 10% of calories, or their usual care with no defined dietary parameters. Smokers on the intervention were also counselled to stop smoking, and those who were overweight were encouraged to decrease total caloric intake and to increase physical activity.

After following all participants for an average of seven years as of February 1982, those on the intervention showed greater decreases in blood pressure, total and LDL cholesterol, rates of smoking and, indeed, slightly fewer deaths from heart disease than those on their usual care. However, total deaths were also slightly greater in the intervention group, driven largely by increased rates of various cancers. Against their own expectations, the study authors concluded that 'the overall results do not show a beneficial effect on CHD or total mortality from this multifactor intervention.'[45]

The 1971 NHLI recommendations had been followed through, without success. There had also been discussion in that report about a possible diet-heart trial on a national scale, but this idea was decided against at the time, primarily out of concern for the practicalities and running costs of such a large trial, which was estimated to run into the hundreds of millions of dollars.[46] Yet 20 years later in 1991, the US National Institutes of Health (NIH) would wind up doing exactly that, as they began a dietary trial on a scale never seen before, or since.

The Women's Health Initiative Randomised Controlled Dietary Modification Trial recruited 48,835 post-menopausal women, 40% of whom were randomly assigned to an intervention diet which aimed to reduce total fat intake to just 20% of calories. These women were also actively encouraged to eat more fruits, vegetables and whole· grains, in accordance with recommendations that had already been enshrined in the USDA's *Dietary Guidelines for Americans* for over a decade to that point, and in the AHA's recommendations for around three. The trial was primarily intended to assess whether such a low-fat diet would reduce the risk of breast or colorectal cancers, but tracked for a range of other issues as well, including risk of heart disease. Participants were followed for an average of over eight years.

The results, published in 2006, could hardly have been more underwhelming. Patients on the intervention ate less fat than their comparison counterparts, and they exercised more. But for all their efforts, they lost an average of less than 1kg of weight, and while their LDL cholesterol was reduced, changes in other markers like triglycerides, HDL cholesterol, glucose and insulin were negligible. More importantly, the low-fat diet also made no significant difference to overall rates of heart attacks or strokes, and for the small subset of women with pre-existing heart disease, their relative risk of further complications was actually increased by 26%.

For a hypothesis as beautiful as that being tested here, these were some ugly findings indeed. This study was supposed to have definitively sealed the deal for low fat, once and for all. But instead, it only raised further questions. Like many of those who had conducted previous trials, the researchers here were at a loss to explain such disappointing results, suggesting that perhaps 'more focused diet and lifestyle interventions may be needed to improve risk factors and reduce CVD risk.'[47]

There was, of course, another possibility, one that was lent further credence by an important observation noted in a paper published in 1999 by Dr Alessandro Menotti, one of the lead Italian researchers for the original Seven Countries study. Menotti had re-examined the original study data and presented updated findings that now incorporated a full 25 years of follow-up information as well. While various foods of animal origin were once again found to be correlated with an increased risk of heart disease, in line with the original study's conclusion on saturated fat, another food category was shown to have an even stronger correlation, namely: sweets, including sugar products and pastries.[48]

If only this second correlation had also been made publicly known back in 1970. If only this second correlation had then been pursued as vigorously and expensively as was the first. (Keys himself was indeed aware of it at the time, but he had instead spent many years arguing against it, and against those who supported it.[49]) Imagine how different the nutrition narrative of today might be, if some of the dietary trials that *have* been conducted over the years were published in a more timely and transparent manner. We might not be so collectively convinced of the killing power of cholesterol, as we have instead been taught to believe. The diet-heart hypothesis might still be seen merely for what it is: a hypothesis, that for all the exhaustive efforts of the scientific community to demonstrate otherwise, appears to remain unproven to this day.

One wonders when more experts might finally come clean and admit that maybe, just maybe ... there was nothing to the diet-heart hypothesis after all, and that maybe more attention should have been paid to the dangers of sugar and carbs instead, as per our previous understanding that had already evolved over the course of our earlier history?

One suspects, sadly, that we may yet be waiting a while.

* * *

The Ministry of Health's current position on low carb for weight loss is to actively discourage consumers from considering it altogether, in spite of the existence of quality evidence that demonstrates a level of benefit and safety that is at least comparable, if not superior, to that of current dietary recommendations.[50]

It is important that the quality of any evidence be considered in an assessment of its value, a measure by which trials typically shine. However, there is also a certain time scale beyond which dietary trials become impractical to conduct. The several-years-long Women's Health Initiative was about as good as it gets in this regard, yet it also cost an eye-watering 700 million US dollars to carry out.[51]

In fairness, the Ministry's definition of 'long term' in its statement is unclear. If, by 'long term' the Ministry means a couple of years or so, then their position on low carb for weight loss is demonstrably false. But if the meaning equates to several more years than the length for which most trials typically run, then we are faced with a dilemma, as the best available data for any defined length of time becomes proportionally weaker, more observational in its nature, as the length of that time period increases.

However, this issue is not exclusive to the case for low carb. The burden of proof in fact does — or at least *should* — apply equally across the board. If the low-carb diet is required to be subjected to this level of scientific scrutiny, then the same should also be true of any other dietary pattern, including those recommended by current guidelines. The minimum length of trials considered for inclusion in the 2020 systematic review on obesity for the *Dietary Guidelines for Americans*, for example, was only 12 weeks.[52] Is that 'long term'?

This really is a key point in the discussion at which different points of view can genuinely begin to emerge. On one hand, it could be argued that observational studies should be taken seriously, because over a sufficiently long period of time, that's all the evidence we have. But on the other hand, it could equally be argued that such evidence is just not strong enough for any given time period, regardless of its availability.

So which way do we go here? In the quest to understand cause and effect processes that can take decades to play out, but with a lack of quality data that spans such extended lengths of time, which fallback approach is more appropriate from a practical standpoint: to settle for observational studies that can cover such timeframes but are still subject to all manner of confounding and bias, or to extrapolate from trial data which is of higher quality but for relatively shorter time periods only?

That's a pretty big question. In more general terms, I cannot even begin to imagine what the best answer to that one might be. I can't even be sure of the right answer in the context of this particular issue. But I do think we now know enough to have at least some idea of the *wrong* answer for this particular issue.

We can see how well one approach has worked in recent decades with the push to recognise low fat as the better option, primarily on the basis of observational studies which paint LDL cholesterol and in turn saturated fat as the villain, but with a lack of support from trial-quality data to back this concept up. We also have the data to demonstrate that our society as a whole has largely embraced this prevailing low-fat advice over the years, and we have all seen the results — or lack thereof — play out as a consequence.

At some level, the establishment does seem to be aware of the failure of the low-fat diet concept as a whole. But rather than admit it outright, we instead see this awareness reflected in the more recent rise of dietary patterns like the Mediterranean diet, which bears all the hallmarks of a typical low-fat diet — fruits, vegetables and grains — modified to now also include certain sources of fats like vegetable oils, in which the types of fats are predominantly unsaturated. The belief that saturated fat causes heart disease, despite a continuing absence of proof from dietary trials, somehow continues to linger on.

This whole situation cannot help but beg the question of the worth of LDL cholesterol as a risk factor for such health conditions. After all, if a so-called risk factor doesn't actually reflect the true level of risk, then how meaningful is it as a marker? Is it even appropriate to call it a risk factor at all? Even if one takes the view that observational studies do have their place in guiding nutrition policy, then it still makes sense to at least consider the strength and consistency of the various known markers of risk, relative to each other, to ensure that we are paying the right amount of attention to the right markers. So what other markers are there, and in that light, how does LDL cholesterol really measure up?

In 1988 Stanford University professor of medicine Dr Gerald Reaven presented a hypothesis that attempted to coalesce a range of metabolic risk factors together into a larger pattern, each of which was already considered consistently representative of risk on its own, but which also provided a further compounding increase in risk when they were found clustered together, as they often tended to be.[53]

Reaven bestowed upon this clustering of conditions the name Syndrome X, and in 2000 he published a book of the same name.[54] Later, the pattern would take on the name of insulin resistance syndrome, after the underlying cause that Reaven considered to be common to each of the presenting conditions, but today it is more commonly known simply as metabolic syndrome.

The list of conditions themselves has evolved over the years, as have the precise cut-off points for diagnosis which, to this day, still vary slightly between organisations.[55] However there is at least now a general agreement that a patient can be considered to have metabolic syndrome if they meet three of the following five criteria:

1. Abdominal or central obesity

Note here the particular focus on the placement of the extra weight, that being specifically around the middle. This emphasis exposes the flaw in relying on the traditional Body Mass Index (BMI) as a measure of risk for individuals, since it is quite possible for fit, muscular athletes to be considered obese by their BMI. A simple measurement of one's waist circumference instead offers a far better guide, even more so when scaled against one's height, to establish a waist-to-height ratio. In a study from 2014, the waist-to-height ratio was found to be significantly more predictive of years of life lost than BMI.[56]

Much of the evidence supporting low carb for weight loss has already been discussed. And, while my own personal experience represents no more than a simple n=1 case study, a mere anecdote, right near the bottom of the pile in terms of grades of quality of scientific evidence, it is still far from unique. When Prof Tim Noakes first began championing LCHF in 2010, he was inundated with so many unprompted letters of support from the public describing their own weight loss success with the diet, that he published a survey of this self-reported data in a paper in 2013.[57]

As we already know, obesity is a plainly and painfully visible concern for so many of us. But it is also the *only* outwardly visible of the five factors behind metabolic syndrome. As depressingly widespread as obesity alone clearly is across our society today, the true scale of the problem is so much greater than merely what we can see.

2. High blood glucose

In his 1988 paper, Reaven proposed that blood glucose levels become dangerously elevated when one's level of insulin resistance becomes too great for one's pancreatic beta cells to be able to compensate through increased insulin secretion, eventually giving rise to chronic hyperglycaemia, or, in other words, type 2 diabetes.[58]

The written history of treating diabetes with low carb goes back even further than that for obesity. In 1798, Scottish surgeon Dr John Rollo published the second edition of his book *Cases of the Diabetes Mellitus*, in which two such cases and their dietary treatment — 'to consist of animal food principally' — were recounted from his time in the military. Both patients, as determined primarily by tracking various measures of their urine, improved over the following months.[59]

A summary of more recent real world examples of treatment of type 2 diabetes with a low-carb diet was published in 2020 by Dr David Unwin, in which 199 diabetic or prediabetic patients at his GP surgery in Norwood, England saw considerable reduction in blood glucose levels by measure of HbA1c, after following the diet for an average of just under two years.[60] These results are backed up by a series of trials having been conducted in recent years, 12 of which were summarised in another 2020 systematic review and meta-analysis, which also found that a low-carb diet tends to produce a reduction in levels of both fasting blood glucose and HbA1c over time.[61]

3. High blood pressure

Widely accepted as a major risk factor for both heart disease and strokes, hypertension has long been considered to be driven by excess consumption of salt. But insulin resistance is also known to encourage the kidneys to retain sodium, thus compounding the salt issue further.[62] So it makes sense that a diet that addresses the issue of insulin resistance might also help with easing hypertension by improving kidney function.

Many of the earlier low-carb trials tracking weight loss also tracked superior reductions in blood pressure. In another example, from 2010, a trial comparing a low-carb diet to low-fat plus the weight loss drug Orlistat, found that the low-carb participants lost only slightly more weight than their low-fat counterparts, but only those on the low-carb diet also reduced their blood pressure at all, allowing many to either decrease their blood pressure medication or even discontinue it entirely.[63]

A wider systematic review and meta-analysis of 14 trials assessing the impact of diet on blood pressure published in 2017 also found that participants on diets lower in either their glycaemic index (GI) or their glycaemic load (GL) — such as a low-carb diet — tended to result in reduced blood pressure versus participants on control diets.[64]

4. High triglycerides

Triglycerides are an effective measure of fat in the blood, produced by the liver from both fructose and glucose in the hours following a meal, the latter as a flow-on effect of insulin which in turn is secreted in order to control blood glucose levels.[65]

It therefore stands to reason that by keeping sugar and carb consumption down, triglyceride levels can also be kept relatively under control. And indeed, this idea is supported by a 2020 meta-analysis of trials assessing the effects of a low-carb diet on various cardiovascular risk factors including triglycerides, which found that low carb can lower levels of triglyceride for up to almost two years.[66]

But what about dietary fat? Just as carbs raise our blood glucose, wouldn't the fat that we eat translate to fat in the blood as well? Not so much. In another trial conducted in 2014, participants began with a low-carb, high-saturated-fat diet, and over the following 18 weeks the carbs were progressively increased, and the saturated fat reduced in such a way that kept total energy intake constant. In the end, the study found that levels of saturated fat in the blood remained fairly constant throughout,[67] a finding which suggests that perhaps we are not so much *what* we eat, as we are what our bodies *do* with what we eat.

5. Low HDL cholesterol

With all the attention paid to LDL cholesterol over the years, it perhaps comes as a surprise that more attention hasn't also been paid to the other kind, the so-called 'good' cholesterol; since, when it comes to metabolic syndrome, there is agreement that low HDL cholesterol features more strongly as a contributing factor and not high LDL. Why might that be?

One important clue to this question dates back to 1986, when an article was published containing findings from the long-running Framingham Heart Study, by which time participants had been followed for 12 years, and where rates of coronary heart disease were compared against both HDL and total cholesterol levels, in combination with each other. The results showed that the incidence of CHD in those with the lowest HDL was around *three times* higher than in those with the highest HDL, regardless of the level of total cholesterol.[68] Since a large proportion of the non-HDL component of the total cholesterol would have been LDL, this would imply that HDL cholesterol is by far the more dominant of the two types when it comes to determining overall risk.

And of course, there is once again no shortage of dietary trials that verify the effects of a low-carb diet on HDL cholesterol levels, many of which were covered in the same 2020 meta-analysis that looked at triglycerides, which also found that low carb can provide steady improvements in HDL cholesterol compared to control diets, for up to two years.[69]

Metabolic syndrome is not at all a controversial concept, nor at this point in time is it even cutting-edge. It simply combines what today may be considered the top five established major risk factors for poor long-term metabolic health outcomes, including heart disease. A list of factors that, notably, does not include LDL cholesterol; a fact which, however inconvenient to some, should not be overlooked.[70] With this wider perspective, there seems little point in continuing to focus on LDL cholesterol to the extent that we currently do, especially when we consider the possibilities that could arise from turning our attention elsewhere, to things like insulin instead.

After all, if there was less reason to fear LDL cholesterol, then there would be less reason to fear saturated fat, since its effects on LDL cholesterol would carry less meaning.

If there was less reason to fear saturated fat, then there would be less reason to fear a high-fat diet as a whole, since the associated increase in saturated fat consumption would also carry less meaning.

If there was less reason to fear a high-fat diet as a whole, then there would be less reason to fear a low-carb diet, since the associated increase in total fat consumption would also carry less meaning.

And if there was less reason to fear a low-carb diet, then maybe we could finally begin to turn the steadily rising tide of chronic metabolic disease that otherwise threatens to overwhelm us all.

* * *

In June 2020 New Zealand's Minister of Health Dr David Clark released the final report of the Government's Health and Disability System Review.[71] The report had been long awaited, with the review itself having first been announced more than two years earlier.[72]

One aspect of the plans proposed by the report in terms of public health was of the general need for the system to focus much more on the population as a whole, not just those who present for treatment; to shift the balance away from treating illness and more towards prevention of illness in the first place. In particular, the report acknowledged the existing burden of non-communicable diseases (NCDs) in this country. 'Looking at current trends, for example increasing rates of obesity, there is an urgent need to accelerate efforts to address these risk factors, and promote interventions to prevent and control them.'[73]

This pivot towards prevention sounds on the surface like a fine idea, but brings with it in my mind two key concerns. First is the fact that New Zealand's overweight population now outnumbers the healthy weight population by a full two to one, and that statistic does not include those with other metabolic health conditions, the combined rate of which has been estimated across various ethnicities in this country to be anywhere from 16% of the population to 39%.[74] For any of these people whose state of health is already compromised, the horse has already bolted. What good does a policy of prevention do for them?

Like it or not, our healthy population is now very much the minority. By focusing on the preservation of health in that minority who still have it, do we not risk losing sight of how best to restore the health of the majority who *don't* have it? Are we to just leave them to their own devices? Do we not, by extension, risk apportioning further responsibility — or even blame — upon these very people for their own illness? As someone who has well and truly been there and lived that, I can personally attest to the sorts of issues that can arise as a consequence of such thinking.

But further to this point, is there any reason why the concepts of prevention and treatment need to be considered separately in the first place? Are these two things really so different? When it comes to low carb, I would argue not. For me, the prevention and the cure have been exactly the same, and my experience is also backed by evidence which suggests that even moderate carbohydrate restriction can still offer further benefits in already healthy people.[75]

My second concern lies with how this proposed preventive focus may be delivered. Various measures have been devised and discussed in recent years, from encouragement of the food industry for healthier formulation of their products,[76] to taxation on sugar and junk food,[77] to more interventions and education campaigns to drive home the existing messaging ever more widely.[78]

But these ideas must surely all be secondary to the need to ensure that the messaging itself is *right*. The effectiveness of the system behind the delivery of the message can only ever be as good as the accuracy of the message itself.

Take a look at any crowd photo that you may find from as recently as the 1970s, and compare it to what you might see in such a photo today. Two generations ago, obesity was an issue that stood out in our society. If you were overweight, you were noticed. Now, conditions like obesity and diabetes are so commonplace that they have almost become accepted parts of the ageing process itself. We resign ourselves to fates so tragically avoidable because they have become so normalised in the face of their sheer ubiquity.

Not only is our current public health crisis too easily written off to general age-related decline, but also to a perceived unwillingness to change on the part of those affected. But in consideration of the latter, nobody *wants* to be fat. Nobody wants to live with any manner of chronic disease. It just doesn't make sense that so many of us, over the course of such a relatively short period of time, could have suddenly become so 'lazy' and 'stupid' with our lifestyle, especially since the data in fact demonstrates a good degree of willingness to change, in support of the messaging that stands currently.

The more likely cause of the problem, on balance, is that the experts of the day simply got that message wrong.

The idea that carbohydrates are somehow such an important part of our diet appears more a legacy of the failed low-fat movement than of any objective assessment of carbohydrates on their own merit. It is simply incompatible with what we now understand about the various dangers of high blood sugar, and the various components of metabolic syndrome through which those dangers begin to manifest.

It is under this wider context of metabolic health as a whole, through which I believe both the scope and the substance of our dietary guidelines should be reconsidered. The management of metabolic syndrome provides a compelling framework around which a more holistic set of recommendations could be developed, one that caters both for prevention *and* for cure. We now know how the right diet can help with addressing a wide range of health issues.[79] The guidelines don't have to be just for healthy people only; they could be made relevant for so many more of us, too.

It may very well be the case, as it was first explained to me as a child years ago, that some of us can and do have a naturally stronger, faster metabolism than others. But it also appears now that, *unlike* what I was told back in the day, those of us with metabolic issues *do* have a tool available to us that can help to address those issues.[80]

I *didn't* have to be fat forever, after all. There *was* something I could do about it.

Is low carb a solution for everybody? Not necessarily, no. But if it has the potential to make more of a difference for an increasing number of people than what is promoted currently, then perhaps this option should be considered further up the list of possibilities than is currently the case.

And just how many of us could it help? In a country of five million where around two thirds of us are overweight or worse, that's well over three million people who might potentially benefit. And even if a figure as small as just 1% of that number were to find success with this approach, then that's still more than 30,000 people directly better off, 30,000 families, schools and/or businesses indirectly better off, and 30,000 potential future long-term patients removed from the public health system, saving that health system millions of dollars of taxpayer funds in the process. Imagine the results if the actual figure of benefit turned out to be closer to 10% of the population, 20%, 40% or more. Such a prospect may not be so far-fetched.

All that needs to happen is for policy to recognise the benefits of this way of eating more than it currently does, to finally forgo our unfounded fears of LDL cholesterol and saturated fat with a view instead towards the bigger picture, where we consider more carefully the apparent consequences of our current direction;[81] to not rely so heavily on weak observational science as we currently do, and to not be so quick to assume that we know as much as we think we know about healthy eating and healthy living, particularly when it comes to the most visible of metabolic issues, that being excess weight and how best to lose it.

Obesity may appear on the surface to be the result of a simple energy imbalance. But when we examine in turn the cause of that energy imbalance, we then see the real root cause of obesity begin to emerge, a root cause also shared by type 2 diabetes, hypertension and dyslipidaemia; *all* of the factors that contribute to metabolic syndrome and, in the long term, any of the myriad of possible adverse health outcomes that can ultimately follow.

Beyond calories alone, what also matters is how well your body manages insulin. If you're insulin sensitive, then the standard advice may suit you just fine, at least for a while. But if you're insulin resistant, then the chances are that something different may be required instead. Ideally, something that both works in the presence of insulin resistance, and helps to address the issue of insulin resistance itself. Something that helps not just to preserve quantity of life, but to improve quality of life along the way also.

And for that, I personally can't think of anything more scientifically valid in theory, more supremely effective in practice, more satisfying for me to eat and more straightforward for me to follow for the foreseeable future, than a low-carb, high-fat diet.

EPILOGUE

May you learn to live without fear
May you be at peace
May your beauty unfold before you
Everything's changed, everything's changed
But I ... am ... home.

—*Devin Townsend Project, 'Truth' (from Transcendence), 2016*[1]

IN 2006, the movie *X-Men: The Last Stand* was released. While a recipient of decidedly mixed reviews by critics, the movie nonetheless stood out to me personally for one of its key plots, around the revelation that a laboratory had developed a cure for the phenomenon of mutation itself.

As someone with an unwanted 'superpower' of my own, I had long related to the characters of the X-Men franchise, as each of them dealt in their own ways with their own unique characteristics that made them all just a bit different from the rest of humanity. As such, I found myself fascinated by the various ways in which different mutants reacted to the news of this so-called cure.

Many were offended by the idea, feeling that their abilities defined who they were, that they were gifts to be embraced, rather than afflictions to be purged. Some believed that their abilities actually made them superior to regular humans, and the fact that human scientists had developed this treatment suggested to them that a larger human conspiracy was at work, to wipe out mutants altogether.

But there were some who felt that their abilities were indeed a burden on their lives. The character Rogue, for example, had the power to temporarily absorb the life energy of others on physical contact, but such contact always left the target person drained; prolonged contact could even kill them. This left her unable to enjoy even the simplest of social interactions such as a handshake, let alone a hug. So she willingly joins the queue to have her power removed, so that she might feel 'normal' for the first time.

To someone already used to the concept, I can imagine that to aspire to normality might seem like a distinctly underwhelming goal. But it's worth understanding the wider contexts from which such aspirations can and do form. For some people, to aim for normality is as lofty a goal as they can possibly conceive, because living with abnormality — no, *sub*normality — is all they have ever known.

As it was for me. But not any more.

The average New Zealand European male is 176.4cm tall and weighs 87kg.[2] As of December 2021, I am 175cm tall and weigh 87kg. Yes, that means a slight re-settlement above what I'd originally achieved, but part of that difference comes from a change of scales in 2017 after the old set broke. In the grand scheme of things, I have remained weight stable.

The jeans I now wear have a waist of 87cm/34 inches, for a total circumference reduction of 45cm, or one and a half feet. Where once my wardrobe was filled with shirts sized at 4XL or 5XL, pretty much everything in there now is either a Medium or Large, depending on the brand. My wardrobe is now an X-free zone.

My blood work has also substantially improved over the years. Since starting low carb, my triglycerides have dropped by a third, my HDL has more than doubled, my blood pressure has normalised and, while I don't have any earlier HbA1c data, that's always been fine for as long as I have been tracking it.

By all of these measures combined, I am about as normal as I can ever hope to be. For the first time in living memory, I am metabolically healthy.

And yet, the physical legacy of my journey remains with me, for those who know where to look.

Since the late 1990s soon after leaving school, I have carried a number of skin tags under my arms and on the back of my neck, although I have since had most of the more prominent ones frozen off. The presence of skin tags on the body is known to be strongly associated with insulin resistance.[3]

Since the early 2010s I have carried a faint rash at the tops of my feet, near the base of the toes, which has never healed. It never occurred to me or to my doctor at the time what a sign such as this could potentially have represented. Maybe I really was a fully-fledged type 2 diabetic at some point? I guess I'll never know now.

It was first pointed out to me a couple of years ago that I have what appear to be two slight but lengthy scars running diagonally across each side of my forehead. It turns out that these are actually oddly placed wrinkles, having developed as a consequence of decades of having to sleep on my sides, for the simple reason that, for the longest time, my sides were the only position in which I could comfortably sleep at all.

And of course, there's a very real scar now running across my abdomen from the surgery. The pain there is long gone at this point, though there is still some degree of numbness that may never completely disappear.

And don't forget the mild turkey neck or the bat wings, either.

But that's all right. These things are just a part of who I am. But considering the bigger picture, where I've come from and where I've been, where I could have ended up versus where I am now?

On the whole, I think I'll be okay.

* * *

I have a pretty decent view from each of the two windows in my bedroom. One looks out over the harbour to the northeast where I catch all the morning sun that I will ever need, while the other offers a panorama of the suburbs to the southeast, with the open ocean resting on the horizon beyond.

One day in early 2019 I found myself staring lazily out the latter of these windows, trying to come up with a way of expressing how my perception of the world around me has changed since having achieved my weight loss goals. And eventually, I came to the conclusion that the way in which I see my surroundings hasn't actually changed at all. What has changed, however, is that I no longer qualify or rationalise those views of the world around me, with views of myself.

To put it another way: I've always been able to derive a degree of enjoyment from various experiences in life, but I haven't always been able to fully appreciate the true value of those experiences solely on their own merits. Every time I used to think to myself, 'that's a nice view,' out the window for example, it would usually only take a few moments for my brain to snap back to reality, and immediately discount the value of having seen that view, because it didn't change the fact that I was still fat.

Here's another example. Say there's a song on the radio that you really like. You might turn it up, start singing along, headbanging away or even dancing to it. We've all been there. 'What a great song!' Until it's over of course, at which point one suddenly remembers. 'Oh yeah, but here I am, still fat.'

Or say you go out to dinner one evening at a fancy restaurant. And it's one of those places where you get what you pay for, so the food is delicious. 'That was such a good meal,' one might think, '... but I probably shouldn't have eaten it, because I'm already fat.'

In one episode of the first season of *Game of Thrones*, Benjen Stark tells Tyrion Lannister that 'nothing someone says before the word "but" really counts.' And I don't think I ever really understood just how right he was until now. Because now, I don't automatically think 'but ...' to myself any more like I used to. Yes, the world around me seems different somehow. But it's not that the world itself has necessarily changed. It's my overall view of that same world that has changed.

Because now, whenever I see, hear, smell, touch or taste something that I like, the memory of that experience is allowed to float around freely in my head for longer, without these other competing thoughts to bring me back down to earth as quickly as before. In effect, the net balance of my very thinking has become more positive, through an increased absence of those negative thoughts.

So now, I can look out the window at home and think to myself, 'that's a nice view,' full stop.

'What a great song,' full stop.

'That was such a good meal,' full stop.

The glasses through which I view the world are just no longer as dark as they used to be. That filtering of old has gone.

I remember a time somewhere around the middle of 2018 when a particular question posted on social media caught my eye. Unlike most things on social media these days — the lolcats, the memes and so on — this one really made me stop and think for a moment. And the question was: 'What is the single greatest benefit of keto or low carb in your life?'

My reply turned out to be surprisingly simple. 'Freedom,' I found myself writing.

Freedom from chronic pain.

Freedom from constant hunger.

Freedom from the usual finger-wagging that I should just eat less and move more. Boy, did that get old fast.

The freedom of choice while clothes shopping. Still wrapping my brain around that one.

The freedom to move and travel in comfort.

The freedom to do something as simple as sleep on my stomach.

The freedom of anonymity. To be able to just stand in a crowd, without standing out.

Freedom.

When I first went public with my own big reveal back in late 2016, somebody asked the question of me directly at that point: 'How do you feel?' And in contrast to the certainty behind the answer to the previous question, on this occasion I actually really struggled to find the words to do this question the justice that I felt it truly deserved. But I think I'd like to finish with a little bit of justice here and now.

So, what emotions do I feel now, at the end of all of this? I've certainly had plenty of time to think about it by this point. There are four in total, but as to which of them I might feel at any given moment, I find that it pretty much varies, depending on the day.

Firstly, there's obviously pride at my accomplishment. Since having lost the weight, I've kept it off so far for a few years now, and counting. I've been able to enjoy a number of new life experiences along the way for the first time, some of which I've written about here, and many of which I would never have considered possible for me beforehand. Achievements great and small, they all count.

There's a bit of anger sometimes, to be fair, that it took so long for me to find something that actually tangibly *worked*. Did that really have to be too much to ask? To have finally found the right information, amidst an absolute sea of ... misinformation, frankly; a lifetime's worth in my case. So many people were so sure of the solution for so long. I've since found that talking about it and, indeed, writing about it, has helped on some of those days.

There's determination, to do my part to ensure that no-one else has to go through what I've been through. To that end, I've completed two certificates while studying part-time with PreKure, one in health coaching in 2019 and the other in nutrition in 2020. I still subscribe to Diet Doctor, in recognition of their work in driving change from the bottom up, and I support the Nutrition Coalition, in recognition of their work to drive change from the top down. Maybe now I have a chance of living long enough to see some of that change actually happen. I hope so.

But ultimately, what I feel is vindication. No one word, to my mind, better describes that feeling of having lived with the constant accusations — some silent, others less so — that I was committing what effectively amounted to a moral crime where my health was concerned, before finally having arrived at the most pivotal and profound of personal truths. A truth that now flies free in the face of what everyone had always assumed of me in the past, and a truth that I hope will continue to sustain me for the rest of my days, whatever those days might bring:

It was *never* my fault, all along.

APPENDIX A: FOOD AND FOOD PLANNING

The shopping list

THIS IS a list of all of the items that have filled my fridge, freezer and kitchen shelves, that have gone into making each of my meals at home across all times of the day, across various days of the week. Every single one of these things I can get from my local supermarket, where I usually go shopping once a week.

It is not meant as a complete list of foods that I could eat (otherwise it might also have included things like asparagus, cabbage, coconut and olives), only those foods which I have personally tried, enjoyed and made work for me. Some things I also eat more frequently than others, mainly because I've found some things more effective for weight loss for me than others. But they have all helped me to varying degrees, at various points in time.

Meat and meat products:

- bacon scraps
- beef steak
- burger patties

- chicken breast or thighs
- lamb chops
- liver
- mince
- pork chops
- salami
- salmon
- sausages
- spam
- tuna

Eggs, dairy and substitute products:

- butter
- cheese
- coconut cream
- cream
- eggs
- sour cream

Fruits and vegetables:

- avocados
- berries (frozen)
- broccoli
- cauliflower
- cherry tomatoes
- courgette
- lettuce
- mushrooms
- spinach
- tomatoes (canned)
- vegetables, soup (canned)
- vegetables, stir-fry (frozen)

Nuts and seeds:

- chia seeds
- macadamia nuts

Flavourings and condiments:

- aioli
- apple cider vinegar
- cranberry juice (low-sugar)
- drinking chocolate (sugar-free)
- dripping
- garlic powder
- olive oil (extra virgin)
- pepper (both black and white varieties)
- salt (Himalayan, iodised, low-sodium varieties)
- seasonings, mixed (Cajun, Tuscan)
- soy sauce
- stock (beef, chicken)
- stevia, liquid (various flavours)
- tomato sauce (low-sugar)
- vanilla extract

Snacks:

- low-carb energy bars

The meal plan (2016)

This is an approximation of the eating plan that I originally developed for myself over the course of my active weight loss journey. See chapter 9 for a breakdown of the recipes themselves.

Breakfast became easy once I'd worked out how best to tolerate eggs: with other things at the same time. Lunch tended to take care of itself, as I could select whatever meat and vegetable-based combinations were going that day at the cafeteria buffet. The real challenge for me was learning how to prepare proper dinners for myself at night, but I got there — or at least, close enough — in the end.

Monday

- Breakfast: cheesy scrambled eggs with sausages
- Lunch: low-carb options from cafeteria buffet
- Dinner: bunless burgers

Tuesday

- Breakfast: cheesy scrambled eggs with sausages
- Lunch: low-carb options from cafeteria buffet
- Dinner: mince with tomatoes, mushrooms and courgette

Wednesday

- Breakfast: cheesy scrambled eggs with sausages
- Lunch: low-carb options from cafeteria buffet
- Dinner: fried salmon and spinach with aioli

Thursday

- Breakfast: cheesy scrambled eggs with sausages
- Lunch: low-carb options from cafeteria buffet
- Dinner: stir-fry with chicken

Friday

- Breakfast: cheesy scrambled eggs with sausages
- Lunch: low-carb options from cafeteria buffet
- Dinner: steak and mushrooms with cauli mash

Saturday

- Breakfast: cherry tomatoes, cheese and macadamia nuts
- Lunch: tuna and cheese omelettes
- Dinner: low-carb takeaways

Sunday

- Breakfast: leftovers
- Lunch: tuna and cheese omelettes
- Dinner: vege soup with spam and cheese

The meal plan (2018)

By the start of 2018 my appetite was well under control to the point where I was no longer feeling the need for breakfast, allowing that habit to come to its natural end once I realised that I just wasn't all that hungry in the mornings any more.

Dropping the breakfast option entirely also meant that I was now eating fewer eggs than before, but they remained as a reserve option for when I felt like something different on any given evening, whether scrambled or as omelettes.

Monday

- Breakfast: cup of warm water with 1 tsp chicken stock
- Lunch: low-carb options from cafeteria buffet
- Dinner: bunless burgers

Tuesday

- Breakfast: cup of warm water with 1 tsp chicken stock
- Lunch: low-carb options from cafeteria buffet
- Dinner: mince with tomatoes, mushrooms and courgette

Wednesday

- Breakfast: cup of warm water with 1 tsp chicken stock
- Lunch: low-carb options from cafeteria buffet
- Dinner: fried salmon and spinach with aioli

Thursday

- Breakfast: cup of warm water with 1 tsp chicken stock
- Lunch: low-carb options from cafeteria buffet
- Dinner: stir-fry with chicken or bacon

Friday

- Breakfast: cup of warm water with 1 tsp chicken stock
- Lunch: low-carb options from cafeteria buffet
- Dinner: steak and mushrooms with cauli mash

Saturday

- Breakfast: cup of warm water with 1 tsp chicken stock
- Lunch: chocolate avocado smoothie
- Dinner: low-carb takeaways

Sunday

- Breakfast: cup of warm water with 1 tsp chicken stock
- Lunch: leftovers
- Dinner: tuna and cheese omelettes

More recently I've been experimenting with a gradual transition away from full lunches as well, with a view to possibly going One Meal A Day (OMAD) on occasion, at least during the week when circumstances allow.

As always though, my hunger dictates how far I go with this. If I'm still hungry at lunchtime, I will still have something. Since the good old cafeteria buffet is sadly no longer operating, I keep a few things on hand at the office such as some salami sticks, cheese, a low-carb energy bar or a bag of macadamia nuts should I feel the need, otherwise I might grab a salad, bunless burger or similar from any of the other nearby shops now and then.

APPENDIX B: WEIGHT LOSS AND BLOOD TEST DATA

Weight loss data

THIS IS a record of my weight for most of the three-year period from 2015 through 2017. The measures weren't taken regularly throughout the journey, just whenever I felt like recording them. Though it seems that I became more and more eager to see where I was up to, as I progressed.

When plotted on a graph, it looks a bit like the second half of a bell curve, or as one observer once described it, 'the most fun part of a roller coaster ride.' It starts off slowly since I began with just walking to work, but things really started to take off once the low carb also got under way.

On the 14th of October 2017 my old scales finally broke, something of an irony considering that it happened after I'd lost the weight and not before. The new digital set that I bought the very next day told me I was 3kg heavier, so there is that discrepancy in my numbers before and after that date due to the change of scales at home. I could have adjusted my earlier numbers up by another 3kg to compensate for the scale change, but I've decided instead to just stick with the numbers I had recorded at the time, with the scales I had at that time.

It hasn't always been plain sailing, though. There was a slight gain during the final months of 2017 when I experimented with a few different, more liberal food choices, and rebounded all the way back up to 90kg on the new scales as a result. But a return to the regular routine in January 2018 saw me revert to 85kg again within a couple of months. Low carb has definitely become my new normal.

The next minor wobble came from the surgery in July 2018, when 1.4kg was removed, but interestingly, my body eventually found its way back to 85kg by the end of that year again, without my having changed anything else at all. It seems that 85kg is just where it wants to be under the usual circumstances.

Those circumstances themselves, however, continue to remain unusual, with the spread of Covid-19. I spent several months working from home during each of New Zealand's 2020 and 2021 lockdowns, which led to further periods of weight creep up to 88kg both times. But upon a return to walking to work again after the first lockdown, along with occasional days of one meal only (at dinner), I returned to 85kg once again within a matter of weeks. My hope remains that the same will happen a second time in due course.

Date	kg	Notes	Date	kg	Notes
03/04/15	137	Started walking	30/07/16	92	
15/07/15	134.5		13/08/16	91	
17/10/15	132	Started LCHF	19/08/16	90.5	
05/11/15	129		26/08/16	90	
22/12/15	123		17/09/16	88	
15/01/16	120		01/10/16	87	
01/02/16	116		15/10/16	86	12 months LCHF
19/02/16	113		05/11/16	87	Travel rebound
11/03/16	110		10/11/16	86	
31/03/16	107.5		19/11/16	84.5	
17/04/16	105.5	6 months LCHF	26/11/16	84	
26/04/16	103.5		11/12/16	83	
05/05/16	102		17/12/16	82.5	
12/05/16	101.5		31/12/16	82	50kg lost on LCHF
14/05/16	101		21/01/17	82	
21/05/16	100.5		28/01/17	82	
22/05/16	100		04/02/17	82	
27/05/16	99.5		11/02/17	82	
11/06/16	98		08/03/17	82	
18/06/16	97		25/03/17	82	Paused tracking
08/07/16	95		01/10/17	82	Resumed tracking
21/07/16	93		14/10/17	82.5	Old scales broke!

Record of author's weight 2015–2017

Blood test history

In 2017 I thought to enquire with my doctor about obtaining a copy of my medical history. This was so I might understand more about where I'd come from in the context of blood measures taken prior to my starting a low-carb diet, with the idea that I might discover other useful markers to indicate progress, in addition to just my weight.

Unfortunately the history does not go back as far as I would like. It has been noted that some earlier data may have been lost as a consequence of the Christchurch earthquakes, which occurred at a time when not all patient records were yet being stored electronically.

The available data prior to my starting low carb may be patchy, but I've made sure to visit my GP annually ever since, and my story continues to strengthen with each passing year. All data since 2016 was gathered in a fasted state; bracketed values have been calculated through various online converters.

November 2009 — hospital visit

- Glucose: 6.0 mmol/L (108 mg/dL)
- Cholesterol: 4.0 mmol/L (157 mg/dL)
- Triglyceride: 1.0 mmol/L (89 mg/dL)
- HDL cholesterol: 1.18 mmol/L (47 mg/dL)
- LDL cholesterol: 2.4 mmol/L (93 mg/dL)
- C-RP: 170 mg/L (1619 nmol/L)

January 2015 — hospital visit

- C-RP: 5 mg/L (47.6 nmol/L)

July 2015 — hospital visit

- Glucose: 5.0 mmol/L (90 mg/dL)

- C-RP: 39 mg/L (371.4 nmol/L)

June 2016 — GP visit, first blood work after starting low carb

- HbA1c: 31 mmol/mol (5.0%)
- Cholesterol: 6.5 mmol/l (251 mg/dL)
- Triglyceride: 0.7 mmol/l (62 mg/dL)
- HDL cholesterol: 1.86 mmol/l (72 mg/dL)
- LDL cholesterol: 4.3 mmol/l (166 mg/dL)

October 2017 — GP visit

- HbA1c: 32 mmol/mol (5.1%)
- Cholesterol: 6.6 mmol/L (255 mg/dL)
- Triglyceride: 0.6 mmol/L (53 mg/dL)
- HDL cholesterol: 2.20 mmol/L (85 mg/dL)
- LDL cholesterol: 4.1 mmol/L (159 mg/dL)

July 2018 — GP visit, taken just prior to surgery

- HbA1c: 31 mmol/mol (5.0%)
- Cholesterol: 6.0 mmol/L (232 mg/dL)
- Triglyceride: 0.6 mmol/L (53 mg/dL)
- HDL cholesterol: 2.27 mmol/L (88 mg/dL)
- LDL cholesterol: 3.5 mmol/L (135 mg/dL)
- C-RP: 1 mg/L (9.5 nmol/L)

September 2019 — GP visit

- HbA1c: 30 mmol/mol (5.0%)
- Cholesterol: 5.5 mmol/L (193 mg/dL)
- Triglyceride: 0.7 mmol/L (62 mg/dL)
- HDL cholesterol: 2.17 mmol/L (84 mg/dL)
- LDL cholesterol: 3.0 mmol/L (116 mg/dL)
- C-RP: 2 mg/L (19 nmol/L)

September 2020 — GP visit

- Glucose: 4.2 mmol/L (76 mg/dL)
- Insulin: 26 pmol/L (3.7 mIU/L)
- HbA1c: 30 mmol/mol (5.0%)
- Cholesterol: 6.0 mmol/L (232 mg/dL)
- Triglyceride: 0.6 mmol/L (53 mg/dL)
- HDL cholesterol: 2.5 mmol/L (97 mg/dL)
- LDL cholesterol: 3.2 mmol/L (124 mg/dL)
- C-RP: 2 mg/L (19 nmol/L)

September 2021 — GP visit

- Glucose: 4.4 mmol/L (79 mg/dL)
- HbA1c: 33 mmol/mol (5.2%)
- Cholesterol: 5.6 mmol/L (217 mg/dL)
- Triglyceride: 0.6 mmol/L (53 mg/dL)
- HDL cholesterol: 2.47 mmol/L (96 mg/dL)
- LDL cholesterol: 2.9 mmol/L (112 mg/dL)
- C-RP: 2 mg/L (19 nmol/L)

APPENDIX C: RECOMMENDED RESOURCES

Further reading

Pure, White and Deadly (1972), John Yudkin
https://www.penguinrandomhouse.com/books/315369/

Protein Power (1996), Michael Eades, Mary Dan Eades
https://www.proteinpower.com/

Good Calories, Bad Calories (2007), Gary Taubes
http://garytaubes.com/works/books/good-calories-bad-calories/

The New Atkins for a New You (2010), Eric Westman, Stephen Phinney, Jeff Volek
https://www.simonandschuster.com/books/The-New-Atkins-for-a-New-You/

Why We Get Fat (2011), Gary Taubes
http://garytaubes.com/works/books/why-we-get-fat/

The Art and Science of Low Carbohydrate Living (2011), Jeff Volek, Stephen Phinney
http://www.artandscienceoflowcarb.com/books/

The Big Fat Surprise (2014), Nina Teicholz
https://thebigfatsurprise.com/

The Real Meal Revolution (2015), Tim Noakes, Jonno Proudfoot, Sally-Ann Creed
https://realmealrevolution.com/real-meal-revolution-book/

What the Fat? (2015), Grant Schofield, Caryn Zinn, Craig Rodger
https://whatthefatbook.com/product/what-the-fat-revised-and-updated/

Always Hungry? (2016), David Ludwig
https://www.drdavidludwig.com/always-hungry-2/

The Obesity Code (2016), Jason Fung
https://www.thefastingmethod.com/books

The Case Against Sugar (2016), Gary Taubes
http://garytaubes.com/works/books/the-case-against-sugar-2016/

Eat Rich, Live Long (2018), Ivor Cummins, Jeffry Gerber
https://www.simonandschuster.com/books/Eat-Rich-Live-Long/

What the Fast! (2018), Grant Schofield, Caryn Zinn, Craig Rodger
https://whatthefatbook.com/product/what-the-fast/

A Fat Lot of Good (2018), Peter Brukner
https://www.fatlotofgood.com.au/

Real Food on Trial (2019), Tim Noakes, Marika Sboros
http://realfoodontrial.com/

The Case for Keto (2020), Gary Taubes
http://garytaubes.com/works/books/the-case-for-keto-2020/

End Your Carb Confusion (2021), Eric Westman, Amy Berger
https://www.adaptyourlife.com/book/

Metabolical (2021), Robert Lustig
https://robertlustig.com/metabolical/

Further viewing

Sugar: The Bitter Truth (2009), Robert Lustig
https://www.youtube.com/watch?v=dBnniua6-oM

My Big Fat Diet (2009), Jay Wortman
https://www.dietdoctor.com/my-big-fat-diet

The Perfect Human Diet (2012), C.J. Hunt
https://theperfecthumandiet.com/

Cereal Killers (2013), Donal O'Neill, Tim Noakes
http://www.cerealkillersmovie.com/

That Sugar Film (2014), Damon Gameau
https://thatsugarmovement.com/film/

Carb-Loaded: A Culture Dying to Eat (2014), Lathe Poland
https://carbloaded.com/

Is Sugar the New Fat? (2014), Nigel Latta
http://tvnz.co.nz/nigel-latta/s1-ep6-video-6060553

The Big Fat Fix (2016), Aseem Malhotra, Donal O'Neill
http://www.thebigfatfix.com/

Fat: A Documentary (2019), Vinnie Tortorich, Peter Pardini
http://fatdocumentary.com

Fat Fiction (2020), Jennifer Isenhart
https://fatfiction.movie/

Sacred Cow (2020), Diana Rodgers
https://www.sacredcow.info/

Further browsing

Real Meal Revolution
https://realmealrevolution.com/

Diet Doctor
https://www.dietdoctor.com/

Ditch the Carbs
https://www.ditchthecarbs.com/

Low Carb Down Under
https://lowcarbdownunder.com.au/

Public Health Collaboration
https://phcuk.org/

Nutrition Coalition
https://www.nutritioncoalition.us/

PreKure
https://prekure.com

ACKNOWLEDGMENTS

This took a long time to write, around five years in total. But then, for most of that time, a book was never the end goal. In fact at first, there was really no end goal to the writing itself at all. For most of that time my writing was simply an outlet for myself, a way of processing my own thoughts, to help me come to terms with what was happening over the course of my journey, without bothering anyone else about the various details of it all.

Being the introvert that I am, I debated for a long time whether or not I felt I could deal with the responsibility of accepting whatever attention I might attract as a consequence of releasing this to the world. It would have been so much easier if the subject matter were literally anything other than myself, fictitious or otherwise.

But of course, it's not.

If you're reading this, then you now know what the answer to that question finally turned out to be. I sincerely hope for your sake as well as mine, that it was worth it.

The very first hat tip that I would like to offer is to Sequoia, for first introducing me in 2018 to the music of Devin Townsend. I ended up listening to far too much of his stuff — mainly the DTP era — while writing a lot of this, and even made the trip to Auckland to watch him perform live in 2019. Along the way, I've also found Devin's own ideas on the creative process itself to be particularly insightful. Thanks, Dev.

The world of publishing was always a mystery to me prior to writing this book, and largely remains so even now. The vast majority of work in this space was led and organised by Martin Taylor of Digital Strategies Ltd, whose expert guidance every step of the way has been instrumental in seeing this project through to its completion. For anyone else finding themselves similarly burdened both with the achievement of having written their story on one hand, and with the uncertainty of what to do with that story next on the other, I cannot recommend Martin's services more highly.

Several others played their part prior to the publishing process as well. I am especially grateful for the fact-checking and preliminary review services of Dr Gary Fettke, Dr David Ludwig, Dawn Ludwig, Prof Grant Schofield, Dr Rod Tayler and Dr Chris Webster. My thanks also to those willing and able proofreaders for their honest feedback on earlier versions of the manuscript as a whole, including Liz, Jill and Rachel, and a whole host more for their thoughts on various individual chapters. You all know who each of you are.

Readers will no doubt have noticed that throughout this book, I have not mentioned the names of any people that I have had any direct dealings with over the years, except for those who are already public figures in their own right. I have also taken care not to name too many companies or brands that weren't directly relevant to the story as it was being told. This was a deliberate decision, made in order to highlight the very personal nature of the story.

Some people have also indicated a preference to remain anonymous anyway, and I am of course respecting their wishes. The rest, however, I would like to fully acknowledge here.

To all of my immediate family, thank you for putting up with me in every respect, both the way I was, and the way I am now.

To Rose and Ralph, thank you for keeping the secret. To Kristin, thank you for noticing. And to Robbie and Sarah, thank you for your invitation to — and your helping me to survive — the Kepler Track.

To Richie, Anna, Dominik, Maya and Rocky, thank you all very much for looking after me while I was out of action.

To all of my work colleagues who encouraged me during the Great Shedding of 2016, thank you for your words of support.

To all of my online low-carb friends, including Janet, Jo, MickiSue, Jean, Ken, Barbara, Marvin, Riolis, Thud, Maeve, Chris, Bev, Jess, Ruca, Tess, Arielle and anyone else that I've missed: thank you all for helping to light the path, and for allowing my real-life friends and family the occasional break from my incessant ramblings along the way.

And to Tracey, my first real-life low-carb friend: thank you for listening, for understanding, and just for being you.

I would also like to express my gratitude to several of those professional figures who I did already name, as well as a few others, many of whom I have since had the privilege of meeting, and all of whom have played no small part in this story — directly or indirectly — as true experts in their field.

To Prof Grant Schofield, Dr Louise Schofield, and the entire PreKure team including Steph, Ulrika, George, Charlie, Sonya, Paula, Carlo, Chris and Glen: thank you all so much for your towering support and encouragement of me and my story. This book would likely not have happened without you.

Also of the faculty, special thanks to Dr Caryn Zinn, for helping to rescue the image of dietitians everywhere in my mind; to Dr Simon Thornley, for helping me to understand both what quality science is and what it isn't; and to Dr Catherine Crofts, for kindly answering my nerdy questions about insulin that I imagine she's heard a million times before.

To Libby Jenkinson from Ditch the Carbs, thank you for your enthusiasm, endless and infectious as it is.

To Dr Rod Tayler, thank you for graciously allowing me the stage for the first time at Low Carb Gold Coast, and then again at Low Carb Denver, the grandest low-carb event of them all.

To Dr Andreas Eenfeldt and the Diet Doctor team, thank you for accepting my original success story, and for your services ever since. Seriously, your video library is pretty much my Netflix these days.

To Nina Teicholz and the Nutrition Coalition, thank you for all your efforts in tackling what must sometimes feel like the hardest job in the world.

To Gary Taubes, thank you for your work in keeping the great nutrition debate alive for the 21st century.

To Prof Tim Noakes, thank you for your courage in the face of it all; and to both you, and Jonno Proudfoot and the Real Meal Revolution team, my sincerest thanks for not just having changed the course of my life, but considering the state that it had reached by 2015, for quite possibly having saved it.

To all of the other researchers, authors, presenters and filmmakers whose works I have also absorbed over the last few years, thank you all for providing further pieces to the puzzle.

To Dr Matthew Hamilton, thank you for having my back throughout the journey and beyond.

To Patrick Lyall, thank you for helping to preserve the symmetry, and to fulfil the dream.

And finally to Rowan Ellis of Body Synergy Gym in Dunedin, from where it all began, thank you for having the good integrity to tell me not what I wanted to hear, but what I needed to hear.

ABOUT THE AUTHOR

Brendan Reid is a former fat broadcaster turned fat software developer, currently based in Dunedin, New Zealand, now minus the fat.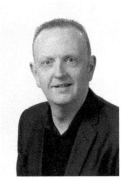

After finally losing more than 50kg (III pounds) in under two years, Brendan's original weight loss success story was featured on Diet Doctor in 2017, and since 2019 he has spoken of his experience at live events both at home and overseas.

Between ongoing work and video game habits, his book *The Fat Ginger Nerd* took around five years to write, and around forty years to live.

https://thefatgingernerd.com

NOTES

Introduction

1. *Bertrand Russell*. (2003, July 11). Wikiquote. https://en.wikiquote.org/wiki/Bertrand_Russell#Proposed_Roads_To_Freedom_(1918)

2. United States Senate Select Committee on Nutrition and Human Needs. (1977, February). *Dietary Goals for the United States*. U.S. Government Printing Office.

3. Yudkin, J. (1972). *Pure, White and Deadly: The Problem of Sugar*. Davis-Poynter, London.

4. Keys, A. (1970). *Coronary Heart Disease in Seven Countries*. American Heart Association, New York, NY.

5. Taubes, G. (2008). *Good Calories, Bad Calories: Fats, Carbs, and the Controversial Science of Diet and Health*. Anchor, 45.

6. Ibid. 5; 51.

7. Harcombe, Z., Baker, J. S., Cooper, S. M., et al. (2015). Evidence from randomised controlled trials did not support the introduction of dietary fat guidelines in 1977 and 1983: A systematic review and meta-analysis. *Open Heart*, 2(1), e000196. https://doi.org/10.1136/openhrt-2014-000196

8. Ibid. 7.

9. *1980 Dietary Guidelines*. (2021, August 24). Office of Disease Prevention and Health Promotion. https://health.gov/our-work/nutrition-physical-activity/dietary-guidelines/previous-dietary-guidelines/1980

10. *Food-based dietary guidelines - New Zealand*. (n.d.). Food and Agriculture Organization of the United Nations. Retrieved November 26, 2021, from https://www.fao.org/nutrition/education/food-dietary-guidelines/regions/countries/new%20zealand/en/

11. *Evidence for the Eating and Activity Statements*. (2021, September 5). Ministry of Health NZ. https://www.health.govt.nz/our-work/eating-and-activity-guidelines/evidence-eating-and-activity-statements

12. *A Picture of Health*. (1993). Ministry of Health Library. https://www.moh.govt.nz/notebook/nbbooks.nsf/0/284859DFA755A63C4C2565D700187296

13. *Tier 1 statistics 2019/20: New Zealand health survey*. (2020, November 18). Ministry of Health NZ. https://www.health.govt.nz/publication/tier-1-statistics-2019-20-new-zealand-health-survey

14. Ibid. 12.

15. Ibid. 13.

16. Ibid. 12.

17. Ibid. 13.

18. Wing, R. R., & Phelan, S. (2005). Long-term weight loss maintenance. *The American Journal of Clinical Nutrition, 82*(1), 222S-225S. https://doi.org/10.1093/ajcn/82.1.222s

1. The Fat Kid

1. Mann, J., & Truswell, A. S. (Eds.). (2017). *Essentials of Human Nutrition* (5th ed.). Oxford University Press, 348.
2. *Aerobics Oz Style.* (2021, August 31). Wikipedia. Retrieved November 26, 2021, from https://en.wikipedia.org/wiki/Aerobics_Oz_Style
3. *Jump Rope for Heart.* (2021, March 8). Wayback Machine. https://web.archive.org/web/20210308102143/https://www.heartfoundation.org.nz/professionals/early-learning-and-schools/jump-rope-for-heart
4. *The food pyramid — shaky science or sound advice?* (2017, March 13). Stuff. https://www.stuff.co.nz/life-style/well-good/teach-me/88284116/the-food-pyramid--shaky-science-or-sound-advice

2. The Escape

1. Barry, L. (2008). *What It Is.* Drawn and Quarterly.
2. *Ghostbusters.* (2021, August 20). Wikipedia. Retrieved November 26, 2021, from https://en.wikipedia.org/wiki/Ghostbusters_(1984_video_game)
3. *Elite.* (2021, September 1). Wikipedia. Retrieved November 26, 2021, from https://en.wikipedia.org/wiki/Elite_(video_game)
4. *Begin.* (2021, August 19). Wikipedia. Retrieved November 26, 2021, from https://en.wikipedia.org/wiki/Begin_(video_game)
5. *Dune.* (2021, April 29). Wikipedia. Retrieved November 26, 2021, from https://en.wikipedia.org/wiki/Dune_(video_game)
6. Whittaker, N., & Moses, R. (1994). *Making Money Made Simple.* Moa Beckett.
7. *Twisted Metal 2.* (2021, September 23). Wikipedia. Retrieved November 26, 2021, from https://en.wikipedia.org/wiki/Twisted_Metal_2
8. *Diablo II.* (2021, September 28). Wikipedia. Retrieved November 26, 2021, from https://en.wikipedia.org/wiki/Diablo_II
9. *Guild Wars.* (2021, August 4). Wikipedia. Retrieved November 26, 2021, from https://en.wikipedia.org/wiki/Guild_Wars_(video_game)
10. *Guild Wars 2.* (2021, August 7). Wikipedia. Retrieved November 26, 2021, from https://en.wikipedia.org/wiki/Guild_Wars_2

3. The Fat Guy

1. Banting, W. (1864). *Letter on Corpulence, Addressed to the Public* (3rd ed.). Harrison & Sons, London, 13.

4. The Moment

1. Knoblich, G., Ohlsson, S., & Raney, G. E. (2001). An eye movement study of insight problem solving. *Memory & Cognition, 29*(7), 1000-1009. https://doi.org/10.3758/bf03195762

2. *Real Meal Revolution*. (2021, August 22). Real Meal Revolution. https://realmealrevolution.com/

5. The Journey, part 1

1. *A Series of Unfortunate Events* (2020, December 1). Lemony Snicket. https://www.lemonysnicket.com/

2. *Real Meal Revolution*. (2018, November 1). Real Meal Revolution. https://realmealrevolution.com/real-meal-revolution-book/

3. TEDx Talks. (2015, May 4). *Reversing Type 2 diabetes starts with ignoring the guidelines* [Video]. YouTube. https://www.youtube.com/watch?v=da1vvigy5tQ

4. Low Carb Down Under. (2014, September 21). *The Art and Science of Low Carb Living and Performance* [Video]. YouTube. https://www.youtube.com/watch?v=GkQYZ6FbsmI

5. McClernon, F. J., Yancy, W. S., Eberstein, J. A., et al. (2007). The effects of a low-carbohydrate ketogenic diet and a low-fat diet on mood, hunger, and other self-reported symptoms. *Obesity, 15*(1), 182–182. https://doi.org/10.1038/oby.2007.516

6. Volek, J. S., & Phinney, S. D. (2011). *The Art and Science of Low Carbohydrate Living: An expert guide to making the life-saving benefits of carbohydrate restriction sustainable and enjoyable*. Beyond Obesity LLC.

7. Westman, E. C., Volek, J. S., & Phinney, S. D. (2010). *The New Atkins for a New You: The ultimate diet for shedding weight and feeling great*. Random House.

8. Schofield, G., Zinn, C., & Rodger, C. (2015). *What the Fat?: How to live the ultimate Low-Carb, Healthy-Fat lifestyle*. The Real Food Publishing Company.

6. The Journey, part 2

1. *Talk:Tom Hiddleston*. (n.d.). Wikiquote. Retrieved November 26, 2021, from https://en.wikiquote.org/wiki/Talk:Tom_Hiddleston

2. Taubes, G. (2011). *Why We Get Fat And What to Do About It*. Anchor.

3. *Cholesterol converter*. (n.d.). Online Conversion. Retrieved November 26, 2021, from https://www.onlineconversion.com/cholesterol.htm

4. *The importance of the fasting TG/HDL ratio*. (2017, July 10). The Science of Human Potential. https://profgrant.com/2016/12/01/the-importance-of-the-fasting-tghdl-ratio/

5. Taubes, G. (2008). *Good Calories, Bad Calories: Fats, Carbs, and the Controversial Science of Diet and Health*. Anchor.

6. O'Neill, D., & Malhotra, A. (2016). *The Big Fat Fix*. The Big Fat Fix Movie. https://www.thebigfatfix.com/

7. *Rowan Ellis - playlist*. (n.d.). YouTube. Retrieved November 26, 2021, from https://www.youtube.com/c/RowanEllis/playlist

8. *Diet Doctor*. (2021, November 17). Diet Doctor. https://www.dietdoctor.com

7. The Rewards

1. Krakauer, J. (1997). *Into the Wild*. Anchor.

8. The Dream

1. Shaikh, S., & Leonard-Amodeo, J. (2005). The deviating eyes of Michelangelo's David. *Journal of the Royal Society of Medicine, 98*(2), 75–76. https://doi.org/10.1177/014107680509800213

2. Teicholz, N. (2015). *The Big Fat Surprise: Why butter, meat and cheese belong in a healthy diet*. Simon & Schuster.

9. The Kitchen

1. Ebstein, W. (1884). *Corpulence and its Treatment on Physiological Principles* (A. H. Keane, Trans.) (6th ed.). H. Grevel, London, 46.

2. *Albert Einstein*. (2003, July 10). Wikiquote. Retrieved November 26, 2021, from https://en.wikiquote.org/wiki/Albert_Einstein

3. *Nutrition information panels*. (2020, August 17). Food Standards Australia New Zealand. https://www.foodstandards.govt.nz/consumer/labelling/panels/Pages/default.aspx

4. Ministry for Primary Industries. (2020, November 16). *How to read food labels*. MPI, NZ Government. https://www.mpi.govt.nz/food-safety-home/how-read-food-labels/

5. Zinn, C., Rush, A., & Johnson, R. (2018). Assessing the nutrient intake of a low-carbohydrate, high-fat (LCHF) diet: A hypothetical case study design. *BMJ Open, 8*(2), e018846. https://doi.org/10.1136/bmjopen-2017-018846

6. Eenfeldt, A. (2021, November 17). *Keto sweeteners - The visual guide to the best and worst*. Diet Doctor. https://www.dietdoctor.com/low-carb/keto/sweeteners

10. The Issue, part 1

1. Blyton, E. (2015). *The Naughtiest Girl Collection 1: Books 1–3*. Hachette UK.

2. *New appointment to support physical activity and nutrition in schools*. (2017, April 13). The Beehive. https://www.beehive.govt.nz/release/new-appointment-support-physical-activity-and-nutrition-schools

3. *Appointment process of Grant Schofield, Chief Education Health and Nutrition Advisor — an Official Information Act request to State Services Commission.* (2017, June 15). FYI. https://fyi.org.nz/request/5736-appointment-process-of-grant-schofield-chief-education-health-and-nutrition-advisor

4. Sboros, M. (2017, October 31). *Does DAA target dissident dietitians with fake news?* Foodmed.net. https://foodmed.net/2017/01/daa-targets-dietitians-with-fake-news/

5. *Dr Annika Dahlqvist, MD – the first LCHF pioneer.* (2019, February 23). WayBack Machine. https://web.archive.org/web/20190223055046/https://foodandhealthrevolution.com/dr-annika-dahlqvist-md-the-first-lchf-pioneer/

6. Ibid. 4.

7. Sboros, M. (2017, October 18). *Dr Èvelyne Bourdua-Roy: Is she Canada's Tim Noakes?* Foodmed.net. https://foodmed.net/2017/10/dr-evelyne-bourdua-roy-canada-tim-noakes/

8. *'Change your diet or you'll die': Low-carb advice lands doctor in hot water.* (2016, November 30). Australian Broadcasting Corporation. https://www.abc.net.au/news/2016-11-30/low-carb-advice-lands-doctor-in-hot-water/8078748

9. Fettke, B. (2018). *Breaking news ... AHPRA drop all charges! #isupportgary.* https://isupportgary.com/articles/ahpra-drop-all-charges-gary-fettke

10. Noakes, T. (2014, February 6). *@ProfTimNoakes.* Twitter. https://twitter.com/proftimnoakes/status/431133258466611200

11. *The Noakes trial.* (2016, October 9). Foodmed.net. https://foodmed.net/the-noakes-trial/

12. Cape Town Live. (2021, September 28). *Tim Noakes trial.* YouTube. https://www.youtube.com/playlist?list=PLPdaIYn6bpO6DG_b5_wAVXf10oniaaJDX

13. Sboros, M. (2020, June 26). *Noakes not guilty! No harm proven, no laws broken.* Foodmed.net. https://foodmed.net/2017/04/noakes-not-guilty-no-harm-proven-no-laws-broken/

14. Sboros, M. (2018, December 12). *Noakes: World watches as HPCSA decides his fate.* Foodmed.net. https://foodmed.net/2018/02/noakes-scientific-medical-world-watches-hpcsa/

15. Sboros, M. (2019, June 14). *Noakes free at last, HPCSA licks its wounds.* Foodmed.net. https://foodmed.net/2018/06/noakes-free-hpcsa-licks-wounds-lchf/

16. Noakes, T., & Sboros, M. (2019). *Real Food on Trial: How the diet dictators tried to destroy a top scientist.* Columbus Publishing.

17. *600+ low-carb & keto success stories.* (2020, January 2). Diet Doctor. https://www.dietdoctor.com/low-carb/success-stories

18. Gudzune, K. A., Doshi, R. S., Mehta, A. K., et al. (2015). Efficacy of commercial weight-loss programs. *Annals of Internal Medicine, 162*(7), 501. https://doi.org/10.7326/m14-2238

19. Stratton, I. M. (2000). Association of glycaemia with macrovascular and microvascular complications of type 2 diabetes (UKPDS 35): Prospective observational study. *BMJ, 321*(7258), 405–412. https://doi.org/10.1136/bmj.321.7258.405

20. Hall, J. E. (2016). *Guyton and Hall Textbook of Medical Physiology* (13th ed.). Elsevier Health Sciences, 990–991.

21. Ibid. 20; 985–987.

22. Ibid. 20; 987–988.

23. Fung, J. (2020, September 30). *Why the first law of thermodynamics is utterly irrelevant.* Wayback Machine. https://web.archive.org/web/20200930082926/https://www.dietdoctor.com/first-law-thermodynamics-utterly-irrelevant

24. U.S. Public Health Service. (1988). *The Surgeon General's Report on Nutrition and Health: Summary and Recommendations.* U.S. Government Printing Office, 45.

25. Foster-Schubert, K. E., Overduin, J., Prudom, C. E., et al. (2008). Acyl and total ghrelin are suppressed strongly by ingested proteins, weakly by lipids, and biphasically by carbohydrates. *The Journal of Clinical Endocrinology & Metabolism, 93*(5), 1971–1979. https://doi.org/10.1210/jc.2007-2289

26. Domb, A. J., Kost, J., & Wiseman, D. (1998). *Handbook of Biodegradable Polymers.* CRC Press, 275.

27. *Dr David Unwin's Sugar Infographics.* (n.d.). Public Health Collaboration. Retrieved November 26, 2021, from https://phcuk.org/sugar/

28. Wasserman, D. H. (2009). Four grams of glucose. *American Journal of Physiology-Endocrinology and Metabolism, 296*(1), E11–E21. https://doi.org/10.1152/ajpendo.90563.2008

29. Erion, K. A., & Corkey, B. E. (2017). Hyperinsulinemia: A cause of obesity? *Current Obesity Reports, 6*(2), 178–186. https://doi.org/10.1007/s13679-017-0261-z

30. Facchini, F. S., Hua, N., Abbasi, F., et al. (2001). Insulin resistance as a predictor of age-related diseases. *The Journal of Clinical Endocrinology & Metabolism, 86*(8), 3574–3578. https://doi.org/10.1210/jcem.86.8.7763

31. Ibid. 20; 997.

32. The DCCT Research Group. (1988). Weight gain associated with intensive therapy in the diabetes control and complications trial. *Diabetes Care, 11*(7), 567–573. https://doi.org/10.2337/diacare.11.7.567

33. Taubes, G. (2008). *Good Calories, Bad Calories: Fats, Carbs, and the Controversial Science of Diet and Health.* Anchor, 400.

34. Fung, J. (2016). *The Obesity Code: Unlocking the secrets of weight loss.* Greystone Books, 4.

35. *Randomised controlled trials (RCTs).* (n.d.). Public Health Collaboration. Retrieved November 26, 2021, from https://phcuk.org/evidence/rcts/

36. Hession, M., Rolland, C., Kulkarni, U., et al. (2009). Systematic review of randomized controlled trials of low-carbohydrate vs. low-fat/low-calorie diets in the management of obesity and its comorbidities. *Obesity Reviews, 10*(1), 36–50. https://doi.org/10.1111/j.1467-789x.2008.00518.x

37. Bueno, N. B., De Melo, I. S., De Oliveira, S. L., et al. (2013). Very-low-carbohydrate ketogenic diet v. low-fat diet for long-term weight loss: A meta-analysis of randomised controlled trials. *British Journal of Nutrition, 110*(7), 1178–1187. https://doi.org/10.1017/s0007114513000548

38. Gardner, C. D., Kiazand, A., Alhassan, S., et al. (2007). Comparison of the Atkins, Zone, Ornish, and LEARN diets for change in weight and related risk factors

among overweight premenopausal women: The A to Z weight loss study: A randomized trial. *JAMA, 298*(2), 178. https://doi.org/10.1001/jama.297.9.969

39. Shai, I., Schwarzfuchs, D., Henkin, Y., et al. (2008). Weight loss with a low-carbohydrate, Mediterranean, or low-fat diet. *New England Journal of Medicine, 359*(20), 2169–2172. https://doi.org/10.1056/NEJMoa0708681

40. Hallberg, S. J., McKenzie, A. L., Williams, P. T., et al. (2018). Effectiveness and safety of a novel care model for the management of type 2 diabetes at 1 year: An open-label, non-randomized, controlled study. *Diabetes Therapy, 9*(2), 583–612. https://doi.org/10.1007/s13300-018-0373-9

41. Athinarayanan, S. J., Adams, R. N., Hallberg, S. J., et al. (2019). Long-term effects of a novel continuous remote care intervention including nutritional ketosis for the management of type 2 diabetes: A 2-Year non-randomized clinical trial. *Frontiers in Endocrinology, 10.* https://doi.org/10.3389/fendo.2019.00348

42. McKenzie, A., Athinarayanan, S., Adams, R., et al. (2020). A continuous remote care intervention utilizing carbohydrate restriction including nutritional ketosis improves markers of metabolic risk and reduces diabetes medication use in patients with type 2 diabetes over 3.5 years. *Journal of the Endocrine Society, 4* (Supplement 1). https://doi.org/10.1210/jendso/bvaa046.2302

43. Foster, G. D., Wyatt, H. R., Hill, J. O., et al. (2010). Weight and metabolic outcomes after 2 years on a low-carbohydrate versus low-fat diet. *Annals of Internal Medicine, 153*(3), 147. https://doi.org/10.7326/0003-4819-153-3-201008030-00005

44. Johnston, B. C., Kanters, S., Bandayrel, K., et al. (2014). Comparison of weight loss among named diet programs in overweight and obese adults. *JAMA, 312*(9), 923. https://doi.org/10.1001/jama.2014.10397

45. Pittas, A. G., Das, S. K., Hajduk, C. L., et al. (2005). A low-glycemic load diet facilitates greater weight loss in overweight adults with high insulin secretion but not in overweight adults with low insulin secretion in the CALERIE trial. *Diabetes Care, 28*(12), 2939–2941. https://doi.org/10.2337/diacare.28.12.2939

46. Bertsch, R. A., & Merchant, M. A. (2015). Study of the use of lipid panels as a marker of insulin resistance to determine cardiovascular risk. *The Permanente Journal, 19*(4), 4–10. https://doi.org/10.7812/tpp/14-237

47. Forsythe, C. E., Phinney, S. D., Fernandez, M. L., et al. (2007). Comparison of low-fat and low-carbohydrate diets on circulating fatty acid composition and markers of inflammation. *Lipids, 43*(1), 65–77. https://doi.org/10.1007/s11745-007-3132-7

48. *Eating and Activity Guidelines for New Zealand Adults: Topical Questions and Answers* (2015, October). Ministry of Health NZ. https://www.health.govt.nz/system/files/documents/publications/eag-topical-qa.pdf, 2.

11. The Issue, part 2

1. *Proposals to revise the Virginia constitution: I. Thomas Jefferson to "Henry Tompkinson" (Samuel Kercheval), 12 July 1816.* (n.d.). Founders Online. Retrieved

November 26, 2021, from https://founders.archives.gov/documents/Jefferson/03-10-02-0128-0002

2. *The food pyramid — shaky science or sound advice?* (2017, March 13). Stuff. https://www.stuff.co.nz/life-style/well-good/teach-me/88284116/the-food-pyramid--shaky-science-or-sound-advice

3. *Eating and Activity Guidelines for New Zealand Adults.* (2021, October 7). Ministry of Health NZ. https://www.health.govt.nz/publication/eating-and-activity-guidelines-new-zealand-adults

4. *Eating and Activity Guidelines for New Zealand Adults.* (2015, October). Ministry of Health Library. https://www.moh.govt.nz/notebook/nbbooks.nsf/0/451DF3E216270666CC257EF0007698F8

5. Marventano, S., Vetrani, C., Vitale, M., et al. (2017). Whole grain intake and glycaemic control in healthy subjects: A systematic review and meta-analysis of randomized controlled trials. *Nutrients, 9*(7), 769. https://doi.org/10.3390/nu9070769

6. Sadeghi, O., Sadeghian, M., Rahmani, S., et al. (2019). Whole-grain consumption does not affect obesity measures: An updated systematic review and meta-analysis of randomized clinical trials. *Advances in Nutrition, 11*(2), 280–292. https://doi.org/10.1093/advances/nmz076

7. Kelly, S. A., Hartley, L., Loveman, E., et al. (2017). Whole grain cereals for the primary or secondary prevention of cardiovascular disease. *Cochrane Database of Systematic Reviews.* https://doi.org/10.1002/14651858.cd005051.pub3

8. Harcombe, Z., Baker, J. S., Cooper, S. M., et al. (2015). Evidence from randomised controlled trials did not support the introduction of dietary fat guidelines in 1977 and 1983: A systematic review and meta-analysis. *Open Heart, 2*(1), e000196. https://doi.org/10.1136/openhrt-2014-000196

9. Department of Health and Social Security (1984). *Diet and cardiovascular disease. Committee on Medical Aspects of Food Policy. Report of the panel on diet in relation to cardiovascular disease.* HMSO, London.

10. Harcombe, Z., Baker, J. S., DiNicolantonio, J. J., et al. (2016). Evidence from randomised controlled trials does not support current dietary fat guidelines: A systematic review and meta-analysis. *Open Heart, 3*(2), e000409. https://doi.org/10.1136/openhrt-2016-000409

11. Hamley, S. (2017). The effect of replacing saturated fat with mostly n-6 polyunsaturated fat on coronary heart disease: A meta-analysis of randomised controlled trials. *Nutrition Journal, 16*(1). https://doi.org/10.1186/s12937-017-0254-5

12. U.S. Public Health Service. (1988). *The Surgeon General's Report on Nutrition and Health: Summary and Recommendations.* U.S. Government Printing Office, 33–34.

13. World Cancer Research Fund/American Institute for Cancer Research. (2018). *Meat, fish and dairy products and the risk of cancer.* World Cancer Research Fund International. https://www.wcrf.org/sites/default/files/Meat-Fish-and-Dairy-products.pdf, 31.

14. Ibid. 13; 16.

15. Zeraatkar, D., Johnston, B. C., Bartoszko, J., et al. (2019). Effect of lower versus higher red meat intake on cardiometabolic and cancer outcomes. *Annals of Internal Medicine, 171*(10), 721. https://doi.org/10.7326/m19-0622

16. *Questions and answers on the Eating and Activity Guidelines for New Zealand Adults.* (2018, February 11). Wayback Machine. https://web.archive.org/web/20180211021324/www.health.govt.nz/system/files/documents/publications/qaa-eating-activity-guidelines-nz-adults-v2.docx, 4.

17. Ibid. 16; 6.

18. *Evidence for the Eating and Activity Statements.* (2021, September 5). Ministry of Health NZ. https://www.health.govt.nz/our-work/eating-and-activity-guidelines/evidence-eating-and-activity-statements

19. National Health and Medical Research Council. (2011, November). *A review of the evidence to address targeted questions to inform the revision of the Australian Dietary Guidelines.* Eat For Health. https://www.eatforhealth.gov.au/sites/default/files/content/The%20Guidelines/n55d_dietary_guidelines_evidence_report_2011.pdf, 7.

20. Ibid. 16; 7.

21. *National health survey: First results, 2017–18.* (2018, December 12). Australian Bureau of Statistics, Australian Government. https://www.abs.gov.au/statistics/health/health-conditions-and-risks/national-health-survey-first-results/latest-release

22. *Health at a Glance 2019: OECD indicators.* (2019, November 7). OECD iLibrary. https://www.oecd-ilibrary.org/sites/4dd50c09-en/1/3/4/5/index.html?itemId=/content/publication/4dd50c09-en&_csp_=82587932df7c06a6a3f9dab95304095d&itemIGO=oecd&itemContentType=book

23. Ibid. 22.

24. Birkbeck, J. A. (1983). *New Zealanders and their diet: a report to the National Heart Foundation of New Zealand on the national diet survey, 1977* (2nd ed.). National Heart Foundation of New Zealand.

25. *A Focus on Nutrition: Key findings from the 2008/09 NZ Adult Nutrition Survey.* (2015, July 8). Ministry of Health NZ. https://www.health.govt.nz/publication/focus-nutrition-key-findings-2008-09-nz-adult-nutrition-survey

26. Ibid. 24; 18.

27. *Food for Health: report of the Nutrition Taskforce to the Department of Health.* (1991). Ministry of Health Library. https://www.moh.govt.nz/notebook/nbbooks.nsf/o/C82E28F4AB1A014C4C2565D7000E1265

28. Ibid. 24; tables B15, B16.

29. Ibid. 25; 303.

30. *Tier 1 statistics 2019/20: New Zealand health survey.* (2020, November 18). Ministry of Health NZ. https://www.health.govt.nz/publication/tier-1-statistics-2019-20-new-zealand-health-survey

31. *Life expectancy.* (2020, March). Stats NZ. https://www.stats.govt.nz/topics/life-expectancy

32. *Health expectancy.* (2020, December 18). Ngā Tūtohu Aotearoa – Indicators Aotearoa New Zealand. https://statisticsnz.shinyapps.io/wellbeingindicators/_w_58284c51/?page=indicators&class=Social&type=Human%20capital&indicator=Health%20expectancy

33. Swinburn, B., & Egger, G. (2002). Preventive strategies against weight gain and obesity. *Obesity Reviews, 3*(4), 289–301. https://doi.org/10.1046/j.1467-789x.2002.00082.x

34. *Dietary patterns and body weight or risk of obesity.* (n.d.). Nutrition Evidence Systematic Review. Retrieved November 26, 2021, from https://nesr.usda.gov/dietary-patterns-and-body-weight-or-risk-obesity

35. *A Series of Systematic Reviews on the Relationship Between Dietary Patterns and Health Outcomes.* (2014, March). United States Department of Agriculture. https://nesr.usda.gov/sites/default/files/2019-06/DietaryPatternsReport-FullFinal2.pdf

36. Ibid. 35; 22.

37. Ibid. 34.

38. Ibid. 35; 19.

39. Ibid. 35; 24, 48, 68, 75.

40. Ibid. 35; 43, 83.

41. *Nutrition - search results.* (n.d.). PubMed. Retrieved November 26, 2021, from https://pubmed.ncbi.nlm.nih.gov/?term=nutrition&filter=datesearch.y_1

42. Ibid. 35; 19.

43. Ibid. 35; 19.

44. Ibid. 35; 19.

45. Ibid. 35; 19.

46. Ibid. 35; 19.

47. Ibid. 35; 235, 270, 307.

48. *Dietary Guidelines 101.* (n.d.). The Nutrition Coalition. Retrieved November 26, 2021, from https://www.nutritioncoalition.us/dietary-guidelines-for-americans-dga-introduction

49. *Eating and Activity Guidelines for New Zealand Adults: Topical Questions and Answers* (2015, October). Ministry of Health NZ. https://www.health.govt.nz/system/files/documents/publications/eag-topical-qa.pdf, 2.

50. *2020 Dietary Guidelines Advisory Committee Systematic Reviews.* (2020, July). Nutrition Evidence Systematic Review. https://nesr.usda.gov/2020-dietary-guidelines-advisory-committee-systematic-reviews

51. Dietary Guidelines Advisory Committee. (2020, July). *Scientific Report of the 2020 Dietary Guidelines Advisory Committee.* U.S. Department of Agriculture, Agricultural Research Service, Washington, DC. https://www.dietaryguidelines.gov/2020-advisory-committee-report

52. *USDA and HHS invite public comments on topics and scientific questions for the 2020–2025 dietary guidelines for Americans.* (2018, February 26). USDA. https://www.usda.gov/media/press-releases/2018/02/26/usda-and-hhs-invite-public-comments-topics-and-scientific-questions

53. Dietary Guidelines Advisory Committee. (2020, July). *Scientific Report of the 2020 Dietary Guidelines Advisory Committee.* U.S. Department of Agriculture, Agricultural Research Service, Washington, DC. https://www.dietaryguidelines.gov/sites/default/files/2020-07/ScientificReport_of_the_2020DietaryGuidelinesAdvisoryCommittee_first-print.pdf, 817.

54. *Media Brief: Dietary Guidelines for Corporate America.* (2020, June 16). Corporate Accountability. https://www.corporateaccountability.org/wp-content/uploads/2020/06/2020.06.16-DGAC-Media-Brief_Corporate-Accountability_Final.pdf, 6.

55. *What is the relationship between dietary patterns consumed and growth, size, body composition, and risk of overweight and obesity?* (2020, July). Nutrition Evidence Systematic Review. https://nesr.usda.gov/2020-dietary-guidelines-advisory-committee-systematic-reviews/dietary-patterns-subcommittee/dietary-patterns-growth-size-body-composition-obesity

56. 2020 Dietary Guidelines Advisory Committee, Dietary Patterns Subcommittee. (2020, July 15). *Dietary Patterns and Growth, Size, Body Composition, and/or Risk of Overweight or Obesity: A Systematic Review.* Nutrition Evidence Systematic Review. https://nesr.usda.gov/sites/default/files/2020-07/DP-dietary-patterns-growth-size-body-composition-obesity%20-%20SR_1.pdf, 73, 78.

57. Ibid. 56; 72.

58. Ibid. 53; 480.

59. Ibid. 56; 72.

60. Ibid. 53; 522.

61. Ibid. 56; 72.

62. Ibid. 53; 484.

63. Ibid. 56; 70.

64. Ibid. 56; 48.

65. Ibid. 56; 70.

66. Institute of Medicine. (2005). *Dietary reference intakes for energy, carbohydrate, fiber, fat, fatty acids, cholesterol, protein, and amino acids.* The National Academies Press. https://doi.org/10.17226/10490

67. Ibid. 67; 809.

68. Ibid. 67; 285.

69. Ibid. 67; 278.

70. Ibid. 67; 275.

71. Ibid. 55.

72. Ibid. 55.

73. U.S. Department of Agriculture and U.S. Department of Health and Human Services. (2020, December). *Dietary Guidelines for Americans, 2020–2025.* https://www.dietaryguidelines.gov/resources/2020-2025-dietary-guidelines-online-materials

74. U.S. Department of Agriculture and U.S. Department of Health and Human Services. (2020, December). *Dietary Guidelines for Americans, 2020–2025, Executive Summary.* https://www.dietaryguidelines.gov/sites/default/files/2020-12/DGA_2020-2025_ExecutiveSummary_English.pdf

75. Ibid. 3.

76. *Eating and Activity Guidelines for New Zealand Adults — Summary of Guidelines Statements and key related information.* (2020, December). Ministry of Health NZ. https://www.health.govt.nz/system/files/documents/publications/eating-and-activity-statements-for-new-zealand-adults-summary-of-guidelines-statements-and-key-related-information-jan_21.pdf

12. The Future

1. Noakes, T. (2017, November 10). *@ProfTimNoakes*. Twitter. https://twitter.com/ProfTimNoakes/status/928625135271194624
2. Brillat-Savarin, J. A. (1994). *The Physiology of Taste*. (A. Drayton, Trans.). Penguin Classics.
3. Ibid. 2; 208.
4. Ibid. 2; 208–209.
5. Ibid. 2; 209.
6. Ibid. 2; 218.
7. Dancel, J. F. (1864). *Obesity, or Excessive Corpulence* (M. Barrett, Trans.). W.C. Chewett & Co., Toronto.
8. Ibid. 7; 44.
9. Ibid. 7; 17, 23, 22, 29.
10. Ibid. 7; 45.
11. Ibid. 7; 64–65.
12. Banting, W. (1864). *Letter on Corpulence, Addressed to the Public* (3rd ed.). Harrison & Sons, London.
13. Ibid. 12; 15, 11–12.
14. Ibid. 12; 16–19, 28–29.
15. Ibid. 12; 22.
16. Ebstein, W. (1884). *Corpulence and its Treatment on Physiological Principles* (A. H. Keane, Trans.) (6th ed.). H. Grevel, London.
17. Ibid. 16; 12.
18. Ibid. 16; 16–19.
19. Ibid. 16; 30, 34–35, 45–46.
20. Osler, W. (1912). *The Principles and Practice of Medicine* (8th ed.). T. McCrae (Ed.). D. Appleton & Co., New York.
21. Ibid. 20; 450.
22. Ibid. 20; 451.
23. Ibid. 20; 451–452.
24. Taubes, G. (2008). *Good Calories, Bad Calories: Fats, Carbs, and the Controversial Science of Diet and Health*. Anchor, 182.
25. Frederick Grant Banting (1891–1941) codiscoverer of insulin. (1966). *JAMA: The Journal of the American Medical Association, 198*(6), 660. https://doi.org/10.1001/jama.1966.03110190142041
26. Ludwig, D. S., & Ebbeling, C. B. (2018). The carbohydrate-insulin model of obesity. *JAMA Internal Medicine, 178*(8), 1098. https://doi.org/10.1001/jamainternmed.2018.2933
27. Ibid. 26.
28. *A Focus on Nutrition: Key findings from the 2008/09 NZ Adult Nutrition Survey.* (2015, July 8). Ministry of Health NZ. https://www.health.govt.nz/publication/focus-nutrition-key-findings-2008-09-nz-adult-nutrition-survey, table 3.2.
29. Huxley, T. H. (2011). Biogenesis and Abiogenesis [1870]. *Collected Essays*. Cambridge University Press, 229-271. https://doi.org/10.1017/cbo9781139149273.009

30. Keys, A. (1953). Atherosclerosis: a problem in newer public health. *Journal of the Mount Sinai Hospital New York, 20*(2), 118–139.

31. Gofman, J. W., Lindgren, F., Elliott, H., et al. (1950). The role of lipids and lipoproteins in atherosclerosis. *Science, 111*(2877), 166–186. https://doi.org/10.1126/science.111.2877.166

32. Yerushalmy, J., & Hilleboe, H. E. (1957). Fat in the diet and mortality from heart disease; a methodologic note. *New York State Journal of Medicine, 57*, 2343–2354.

33. Yudkin, J. (1957). Diet and coronary thrombosis: hypothesis and fact. *The Lancet, 270*(6987), 155–162. https://doi.org/10.1016/s0140-6736(57)90614-1

34. Keys, A. (1957). Diet and the epidemiology of coronary heart disease. *Journal of the American Medical Association, 164*(17), 1912. https://doi.org/10.1001/jama.1957.62980170024007e

35. Teicholz, N. (2015). *The Big Fat Surprise: Why butter, meat and cheese belong in a healthy diet.* Simon & Schuster, 32–33.

36. Central Committee for Medical and Community Program of the American Heart Association. (1961). Dietary fat and its relation to heart attacks and strokes. *JAMA, 175*(5), 389–391. https://doi.org/10.1001/jama.1961.63040050001011

37. Keys, A. (1970). *Coronary Heart Disease in Seven Countries.* American Heart Association, New York, NY.

38. Ibid. 37; 191–194.

39. National Heart and Lung Institute. (1971). *Arteriosclerosis: A Report by the National Heart and Lung Institute Task Force on Arteriosclerosis.* Dept of Health, Education, and Welfare publication (NIH) 72–137. Washington, DC, National Institutes of Health. Vol 1, 20–21.

40. Woodhill, J. M., Palmer, A. J., Leelarthaepin, B., et al. (1978). Low fat, low cholesterol diet in secondary prevention of coronary heart disease. *Advances in Experimental Medicine and Biology,* 317–330. https://doi.org/10.1007/978-1-4684-0967-3_18

41. Ramsden, C. E., Zamora, D., Leelarthaepin, B., et al. (2013). Use of dietary linoleic acid for secondary prevention of coronary heart disease and death: Evaluation of recovered data from the Sydney diet heart study and updated meta-analysis. *BMJ, 346*, e8707. https://doi.org/10.1136/bmj.e8707

42. Frantz, I. D., Dawson, E. A., Ashman, P. L., et al. (1989). Test of effect of lipid lowering by diet on cardiovascular risk; the Minnesota coronary survey. *Arteriosclerosis: An Official Journal of the American Heart Association, Inc, 9*(1), 129–135. https://doi.org/10.1161/01.atv.9.1.129

43. Ibid. 24; 38.

44. Ramsden, C. E., Zamora, D., Majchrzak-Hong, S., et al. (2016). Re-evaluation of the traditional diet-heart hypothesis: Analysis of recovered data from Minnesota coronary experiment (1968–73). *BMJ,* i1246. https://doi.org/10.1136/bmj.i1246

45. Multiple Risk Factor Intervention Trial research group. (1982). Multiple risk factor intervention trial: risk factor changes and mortality results. *JAMA: The Journal of the American Medical Association, 248*(12), 1465–1477. https://doi.org/10.1001/jama.1982.03330120023025

46. Ibid. 39.

47. Howard, B. V., Van Horn, L., Hsia, J., et al. (2006). Low-fat dietary pattern and risk of cardiovascular disease. *JAMA, 295*(6), 655. https://doi.org/10.1001/jama.295.6.655

48. Menotti, A., Kromhout, D., Blackburn, H., et al. (1999). Food intake patterns and 25-year mortality from coronary heart disease: Cross-cultural correlations in the Seven Countries Study. *European Journal of Epidemiology, 15*(6), 507–515. https://doi.org/10.1023/a:1007529206050

49. Ibid. 35; 42–43.

50. Castellana, M., Conte, E., Cignarelli, A., et al. (2019). Efficacy and safety of very low calorie ketogenic diet (VLCKD) in patients with overweight and obesity: A systematic review and meta-analysis. *Reviews in Endocrine and Metabolic Disorders, 21*(1), 5–16. https://doi.org/10.1007/s11154-019-09514-y

51. Ibid. 24; 74.

52. 2020 Dietary Guidelines Advisory Committee, Dietary Patterns Subcommittee. (2020, July 15). *Dietary Patterns and Growth, Size, Body Composition, and/or Risk of Overweight or Obesity: A Systematic Review.* Nutrition Evidence Systematic Review. https://nesr.usda.gov/sites/default/files/2020-07/DP-dietary-patterns-growth-size-body-composition-obesity%20-%20SR_1.pdf, 72.

53. Reaven, G. M. (1988). Role of insulin resistance in human disease. *Diabetes, 37*(12), 1595–1607. https://doi.org/10.2337/diab.37.12.1595

54. Reaven, G. M. (2000). *Syndrome X: Overcoming the Silent Killer That Can Give You a Heart Attack.* Simon & Schuster.

55. Grundy, S. M., Brewer, H. B., Cleeman, J. I., et al. (2004). Definition of metabolic syndrome. *Circulation, 109*(3), 433–438. https://doi.org/10.1161/01.cir.0000111245.75752.c6

56. Ashwell, M., Mayhew, L., Richardson, J., et al. (2014). Waist-to-Height ratio is more predictive of years of life lost than body mass index. *PLoS ONE, 9*(9), e103483. https://doi.org/10.1371/journal.pone.0103483

57. Noakes, T. D. (2013). Low-carbohydrate and high-fat intake can manage obesity and associated conditions: Occasional survey. *South African Medical Journal, 103*(11), 826. https://doi.org/10.7196/samj.7302

58. Ibid. 53.

59. Rollo, J. (1798). *Cases of the Diabetes Mellitus* (2nd ed.). T. Gillet, London.

60. Unwin, D., Khalid, A. A., Unwin, J., et al. (2020). Insights from a general practice service evaluation supporting a lower carbohydrate diet in patients with type 2 diabetes mellitus and prediabetes: A secondary analysis of routine clinic data including HbA1c, weight and prescribing over 6 years. *BMJ Nutrition, Prevention & Health, 3*(2), 285–294. https://doi.org/10.1136/bmjnph-2020-000072

61. Yuan, X., Wang, J., Yang, S., et al. (2020). Effect of the ketogenic diet on glycemic control, insulin resistance, and lipid metabolism in patients with T2DM: A systematic review and meta-analysis. *Nutrition & Diabetes, 10*(1). https://doi.org/10.1038/s41387-020-00142-z

62. Horita, S., Seki, G., Yamada, H., et al. (2011). Insulin resistance, obesity, hypertension, and renal sodium transport. *International Journal of Hypertension, 2011*, 1–8. https://doi.org/10.4061/2011/391762

63. Yancy, W. S., Westman, E. C., McDuffie, J. R., et al. (2010). A randomized trial of a low-carbohydrate diet vs Orlistat plus a low-fat diet for weight loss. *Archives of Internal Medicine, 170*(2), 136. https://doi.org/10.1001/archinternmed.2009.492

64. Evans, C. E., Greenwood, D. C., Threapleton, D. E., et al. (2017). Glycemic index, glycemic load, and blood pressure: A systematic review and meta-analysis of randomized controlled trials. *The American Journal of Clinical Nutrition, 105*(5), 1176–1190. https://doi.org/10.3945/ajcn.116.143685

65. Sanders, F. W., & Griffin, J. L. (2015). De Novo lipogenesis in the liver in health and disease: More than just a shunting yard for glucose. *Biological Reviews, 91*(2), 452–468. https://doi.org/10.1111/brv.12178

66. Dong, T., Guo, M., Zhang, P., et al. (2020). The effects of low-carbohydrate diets on cardiovascular risk factors: A meta-analysis. *PLoS ONE, 15*(1), e0225348. https://doi.org/10.1371/journal.pone.0225348

67. Volk, B. M., Kunces, L. J., Freidenreich, D. J., et al. (2014). Effects of step-wise increases in dietary carbohydrate on circulating saturated fatty acids and palmitoleic acid in adults with metabolic syndrome. *PLoS ONE, 9*(11), e113605. https://doi.org/10.1371/journal.pone.0113605

68. Castelli, W. P. (1986). Incidence of coronary heart disease and lipoprotein cholesterol levels. *JAMA, 256*(20), 2835. https://doi.org/10.1001/jama.1986.03380200073024

69. Ibid. 66.

70. Ravnskov, U., De Lorgeril, M., Diamond, D. M., et al. (2018). LDL-C does not cause cardiovascular disease: A comprehensive review of the current literature. *Expert Review of Clinical Pharmacology, 11*(10), 959–970. https://doi.org/10.1080/17512433.2018.1519391

71. *Final report / Pūrongo whakamutunga.* (2020, June 16). New Zealand Health and Disability System Review. https://systemreview.health.govt.nz/final-report

72. *Major review of health system launched.* (2018, May 29). The Beehive. https://www.beehive.govt.nz/release/major-review-health-system-launched

73. *Final report / Pūrongo whakamutunga.* (2020, March). New Zealand Health and Disability System Review. https://systemreview.health.govt.nz/assets/Uploads/hdsr/health-disability-system-review-final-report.pdf, 86.

74. Gentles, D., Metcalf, P., Dyall, L., et al. (2007). Metabolic syndrome prevalence in a multicultural population in Auckland, New Zealand. *The New Zealand Medical Journal, 120*(1248), U2399. https://pubmed.ncbi.nlm.nih.gov/17277815

75. Harvey, C. J., Schofield, G. M., Zinn, C., et al. (2019). Low-carbohydrate diets differing in carbohydrate restriction improve cardiometabolic and anthropometric markers in healthy adults: A randomised clinical trial. *PeerJ, 7*, e6273. https://doi.org/10.7717/peerj.6273

76. *Food Industry Taskforce on Addressing Factors Contributing to Obesity.* (2018, December 20). Ministry of Health NZ. https://www.health.govt.nz/system/files/documents/pages/food-industry-taskforce-final-report.pdf

77. *Implications of a sugar tax in New Zealand: Incidence and effectiveness.* (2017, February 3). The Treasury New Zealand. https://www.treasury.govt.nz/publications/wp/implications-sugar-tax-new-zealand-incidence-and-effectiveness-html

78. *Nutrition and physical activity*. (2020, June 4). HPA - Health Promotion Agency. https://www.hpa.org.nz/programme/nutrition-and-physical-activity

79. Hyde, P. N., Sapper, T. N., Crabtree, C. D., et al. (2019). Dietary carbohydrate restriction improves metabolic syndrome independent of weight loss. *JCI Insight, 4*(12). https://doi.org/10.1172/jci.insight.128308

80. Ebbeling, C. B., Feldman, H. A., Klein, G. L., et al. (2018). Effects of a low carbohydrate diet on energy expenditure during weight loss maintenance: Randomized trial. *BMJ*, k4583. https://doi.org/10.1136/bmj.k4583

81. Astrup, A., Magkos, F., Bier, D. M., et al. (2020). Saturated fats and health: A reassessment and proposal for food-based recommendations. *Journal of the American College of Cardiology, 76*(7), 844–857. https://doi.org/10.1016/j.jacc.2020.05.077

Epilogue

1. Devin Townsend Project. (2016, September 9). 'Truth'. On *Transcendence* [CD]. HevyDevy Records.

2. *Tier 1 statistics 2019/20: New Zealand health survey*. (2020, November 18). Ministry of Health NZ. https://www.health.govt.nz/publication/tier-1-statistics-2019-20-new-zealand-health-survey

3. Tamega, A., Aranha, A. M., Guiotoku, M. M., et al. (2010). Associação entre acrocórdons e resistência à insulina [Association between skin tags and insulin resistance]. *Anais brasileiros de dermatologia, 85*(1), 25–31. https://doi.org/10.1590/s0365-05962010000100003

CPSIA information can be obtained
at www.ICGtesting.com
Printed in the USA
LVHW040844180322
713694LV00002B/136